Aging and Critical Care

Editor

SONYA R. HARDIN

CRITICAL CARE NURSING CLINICS OF NORTH AMERICA

www.ccnursing.theclinics.com

Consulting Editor
JAN FOSTER

March 2014 • Volume 26 • Number 1

ELSEVIER

1600 John F. Kennedy Boulevard ● Suite 1800 ● Philadelphia, Pennsylvania, 19103-2899

http://www.theclinics.com

CRITICAL CARE NURSING CLINICS OF NORTH AMERICA Volume 26, Number 1
March 2014 ISSN 0899-5885, ISBN-13: 978-0-323-26092-3

Editor: Kerry Holland
Developmental Editor: Stephanie Carter

Photocopying
Single photocopies of single articles may be made for personal use as allowed by national copyright laws. Permission of the Publisher and payment of a fee is required for all other photocopying, including multiple or systematic copying, copying for advertising or promotional purposes, resale, and all forms of document delivery. Special rates are available for educational institutions that wish to make photocopies for non-profit educational classroom use. For information on how to seek permission visit www.elsevier.com/permissions or call: (+44) 1865 843830 (UK)/(+1) 215 239 3804 (USA).

Derivative Works
Subscribers may reproduce tables of contents or prepare lists of articles including abstracts for internal circulation within their institutions. Permission of the Publisher is required for resale or distribution outside the institution. Permission of the Publisher is required for all other derivative works, including compilations and translations (please consult www.elsevier.com/permissions).

Electronic Storage or Usage
Permission of the Publisher is required to store or use electronically any material contained in this periodical, including any article or part of an article (please consult www.elsevier.com/permissions). Except as outlined above, no part of this publication may be reproduced, stored in a retrieval system or transmitted in any form or by any means, electronic, mechanical, photocopying, recording or otherwise, without prior written permission of the Publisher.

Notice
No responsibility is assumed by the Publisher for any injury and/or damage to persons or property as a matter of products liability, negligence or otherwise, or from any use or operation of any methods, products, instructions or ideas contained in the material herein. Because of rapid advances in the medical sciences, in particular, independent verification of diagnoses and drug dosages should be made.

Although all advertising material is expected to conform to ethical (medical) standards, inclusion in this publication does not constitute a guarantee or endorsement of the quality or value of such product or of the claims made of it by its manufacturer.

Critical Care Nursing Clinics of North America (ISSN 0899-5885) is published quarterly by Elsevier Inc., 360 Park Avenue South, New York, NY 10010-1710. Months of issue are March, June, September, and December. Business and Editorial Offices: 1600 John F. Kennedy Blvd., Suite 1800, Philadelphia, PA 19103-2899. Periodicals postage paid at New York, NY and additional mailing offices. Subscription prices are $150.00 per year for US individuals, $328.00 per year for US institutions, $80.00 per year for US students and residents, $200.00 per year for Canadian individuals, $412.00 per year for Canadian institutions, $230.00 per year for international individuals, $412.00 per year for international institutions and $115.00 per year for Canadian and international students/residents. To receive student/resident rate, orders must be accompanied by name of affiliated institution, data of term, and the *signature* of program/residency coordinator on institution letterhead. Orders will be billed at individual rate until proof of status is received. Foreign air speed delivery is included in all *Clinics* subscription prices. All prices are subject to change without notice. **POSTMASTER:** Send address changes to *Critical Care Nursing Clinics of North America*, Elsevier Health Sciences Division, Subscription Customer Service, 3251 Riverport Lane, Maryland Heights, MO 63043. **Customer Service: 1-800-654-2452 (US and Canada); 314-447-8871 (outside US and Canada). Fax: 314-447-8029. E-mail: JournalsCustomerService-usa@elsevier.com (for print support) and JournalsOnlineSupport-usa@elsevier.com (for online support).**

Reprints. For copies of 100 or more of articles in this publication, please contact the Commercial Reprints Department, Elsevier Inc., 360 Park Avenue South, New York, New York, 10010-1710; Tel.: 212-633-3874, Fax: 212-633-3820, and E-mail: reprints@elsevier.com.

Critical Care Nursing Clinics of North America is covered in *MEDLINE/PubMed (Index Medicus), International Nursing Index, Nursing Citation Index, Cumulative Index to Nursing and Allied Health Literature,* and *RNdex Top 100.*

Printed and bound by CPI Group (UK) Ltd, Croydon, CR0 4YY

Contributors

CONSULTING EDITOR

JAN FOSTER, PhD, RN, CNS
College of Nursing, Texas Woman's University, Houston, Texas

EDITOR

SONYA R. HARDIN, PhD, RN, CCRN, NP-C
Professor, College of Nursing, East Carolina University, Greenville, North Carolina

AUTHORS

KATHERYNE TIFUH AMBA, MSN, CCRN, ACNP-BC, PhD (C)
Acute Care Nurse Practitioner, Department of Neurosurgery, Barnes Jewish Hospital, St Louis, Missouri

LINDA BELL, RN, MSN
Clinical Practice Specialist, Technology-Based Learning, American Association of Critical Care Nurses, Aliso Viejo, California

BRYAN BOLING, RN, CCRN, CEN
Cardiothoracic Vascular Intensive Care Unit, University of Kentucky Hospital, Lexington, Kentucky

JOAN E. DACHER, PhD, MS, BS, GNP
Professor of Nursing, Director Doctor of Nursing Science Program, Department of Nursing, The Sage Colleges, Troy, New York

LESLIE L. DAVIS, PhD, RN, ANP-BC, FAANP, FAHA
Assistant Professor of Nursing, School of Nursing, University of North Carolina, Greensboro, North Carolina

ROSE ANN DIMARIA-GHALILI, PhD, RN, CNSC
Associate Professor of Nursing, Doctoral Nursing Department, College of Nursing and Health Professions, Drexel University, Philadelphia, Pennsylvania

DELIA E. FREDERICK, MSN, RN
Doctoral Student in Nursing Science, School of Nursing, The University of North Carolina at Greensboro, Oak Street, Franklin, North Carolina

BETHANY GENTLEMAN, MS, GNP-BC
Private Practice, Hamilton, Massachusetts

SONYA R. HARDIN, PhD, RN, CCRN, NP-C
Professor, College of Nursing, East Carolina University, Greenville, North Carolina

LAURIE S. HARTMAN, DNP, RN, ACNP-BC
Clinical Assistant Professor, Director of Advanced Practice Nursing, University of
Michigan Hospitals and Health System, University of Michigan School of Nursing,
Ann Arbor, Michigan

ROBERTA KAPLOW, APRN-CCNS, PhD, AOCNS, CCRN
Oncology Clinical Nurse Specialist, Department of Oncology, Emory University Hospital,
Atlanta, Georgia

HELEN W. LACH, PhD, RN, GCNS-BC
Associate Professor, Saint Louis University School of Nursing, St Louis, Missouri

KRISTINE M. L'ECUYER, PhD(c), RN, CCNS, CNL
Associate Professor, Saint Louis University School of Nursing, St Louis, Missouri

CAMILLE LINEBERRY, MSN, ACNP-BC
Department of Anesthesiology and Critical Care, Memorial Sloan Kettering Cancer
Center, New York, New York

REBECCA A. LORENZ, PhD, RN
Associate Professor, Saint Louis University School of Nursing, St Louis, Missouri

MICHELE NICOLO, MS, RD, CDE, CNSD, LDN
Clinical Dietitian Specialist, Clinical Nutrition Support Services, Hospital of the University
of Pennsylvania, Philadelphia, Pennsylvania

MARY SEBASTIAN, MHA, BSN, CNML
Orientation and Training Coordinator, Nursing Education and Research Department,
University of Louisville Hospital, Louisville, Kentucky

MARK SPIVAK, BSN, RN, CEN
Emergency Department Advanced Practice Educator, Nursing Education and Research
Department, University of Louisville Hospital, Louisville, Kentucky

DEBORAH E. STEIN, MSN, ACNP-BC, CCRN
Department of Anesthesiology and Critical Care, Memorial Sloan Kettering Cancer
Center, New York, New York

LAURA M. STRUBLE, PhD, RN, GNP-BC
Clinical Assistant Professor, Division of Acute, Critical and Long-Term Care, University of
Michigan School of Nursing, Ann Arbor, Michigan

BARBARA J. SULLIVAN, PhD, RN, APRN-BC, NP
Clinical Assistant Professor, Division of Acute, Critical and Long-Term Care, University of
Michigan School of Nursing, Ann Arbor, Michigan

MANDI WALKER, MSN, RN-BC, CCRN
Critical Care Advanced Practice Educator, Nursing Education and Research Department,
University of Louisville Hospital, Louisville, Kentucky

Contents

adult is often complex because of preexisting risk factors (malnutrition, unintentional weight loss, frailty, and dehydration) as well as intensive care unit–related challenges (catabolism, eating and feeding, end-of-life care). This article highlights the challenges of managing nutrition and hydration in the critically ill older adult, reviews assessment principles, and offers strategies for optimizing nutrition and hydration.

The elderly are vulnerable to developing sepsis due to functional and immune changes, and frequent instrumentation and contact with the health care system. Those infected often present with nonspecific complaints and are at risk for underrecognition and undertreatment, with greater likelihood of rapid progression to severe sepsis and septic shock; however, they often respond well to early, organized, and aggressive interventions. Survivors may not return to baseline level of function and may require long-term care facilities after discharge from the hospital. Patient and family preferences for goals of care should be explored as early as possible and incorporated into treatment plans.

This article discusses selected cardiovascular conditions that nurses encounter when caring for elders hospitalized in the intensive care unit. Physiologic changes that predispose elders to these conditions, typical signs and symptoms, common diagnostic tests, and evidence-based treatment for this population are included. The implications for nursing care of critically ill elders who have these conditions are also discussed.

This article elicits why critical care nurses need to become aware of the pulmonary issues of older adults. The population of older adults is increasing. Older adults undergo anatomic and physiologic changes of the protective mechanisms of the pulmonary system. These changes alter the rate and effort of breathing. Speech is slowed because of expiratory strength effort. Cognition changes may be the only indication of impaired oxygenation. Bedside nursing care provides protection from pulmonary complications. Health behaviors of smoking cessation, oral hygiene, and exercise promote pulmonary health even in older adults.

Renal issues are among the most commonly encountered complications in the intensive care unit, increasing mortality, morbidity, and health care costs. Older adult patients face an increased risk because of several factors, including the normal effects of aging and a higher rate of comorbid conditions that may affect kidney function. This article describes the classification of renal dysfunction, the effects of aging on kidney function, as well as additional risk factors, management strategies, and outcomes in the older adult population.

Critical illness can impose immobility in older patients, resulting in loss of strength and functional ability. Many factors contribute to immobility, including patients' medical conditions, medical devices and equipment, nutrition, use of restraint, and staff priorities. Early mobilization reduces the impact of immobility and improves outcomes for older patients. Several important components make up successful mobility programs, including good patient assessment, a core set of interventions, and use of the inter-professional health care team. Nurses can lead in improving the mobilization of older critical care patients, thus reducing clinical risk in this vulnerable population.

An astounding 30% to 50% of older patients who are hospitalized for a medical condition also have a psychiatric disorder. The intent of this article is to prepare acute care nurses to meet the mental health needs of older adults with a critical illness and prevent untoward sequelae of medical events. The authors discuss the importance of baseline assessment data, issues related to informed consent, manifestations of common psychiatric disorders that may be seen in older adults in the acute care setting, as well as strategies to improve patient outcomes.

Several neurologic conditions are commonly seen with elderly adults in the critical care area. This article addresses a common neurologic condition commonly seen in elderly adults: delirium.

This article describes the pathophysiologic changes that occur with aging as they relate to cancer and cytotoxic therapies, implications related to drug therapy, and complications of treatment modalities as they relate to older persons with cancer who may potentially be admitted to the intensive care unit. Knowledge of these issues is essential for health care providers, so that they can face the complex challenges and optimize the outcomes of critically ill older persons with cancer.

Palliative care is emerging as an alternative care paradigm for critically ill older patients in the critical care setting. Critical care nurses are well positioned to take on a leadership role in reconceptualizing care in the critical care unit, and creating the space and opportunity for palliative care. This article provides information on the practice of palliative care with critically ill older adults along with evidence-based content and resources, allowing critical care nurses to advocate for palliative care in their own work environments accompanied by the necessary resources that will support efficient implementation.

CRITICAL CARE NURSING
CLINICS OF NORTH AMERICA

RELATED INTEREST

Geriatric Medicine, November 2011
Successful Aging
Jeremy D. Walston, *Editor*

DOWNLOAD
Free App!

Review Articles
THE CLINICS

NOW AVAILABLE FOR YOUR iPhone and iPad

Preface

Caring for Older Adults in Critical Care

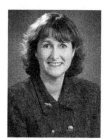

Sonya R. Hardin, PhD, RN, CCRN, NP-C
Editor

This issue of *Critical Care Nursing Clinics of North America* has been designed to focus on the care of the older adult. The proportion of older adults from the total intensive care unit (ICU) population is high. The number of older adults is expected to exceed that of the young by the year 2050; therefore, critical care nurses can expect to see increasing numbers in their units. With advancing age, older adults present with preexisting comorbidities and are at greater risk for mortality, especially if the ICU patient is older than 75.

Fourteen articles have been compiled on the care of older adults in critical care. While not all issues seen in older adults are addressed, major areas of subject matter are presented that will be useful as a review for some and may be new information for others. The first article is by Linda Bell and discusses the epidemiology of acute and critical illness in older adults. She points out that with an extended lifespan, disability rates in older adults have not changed; they are living longer with disabilities that affect their quality of life and complicate acute and critical illness. Individuals admitted to our units often face physiological changes, associated with aging, that increase their risk of mortality. Therefore, the second article in this issue is written by Mandi Walker, Mark Spivak, and Mary Sebastian. A key message in this article is that consideration should be given when addressing the patients' specific needs regarding the systemic changes experienced in aging. Each major body system presents its own unique challenges; therefore, information on changes that occur with aging is presented.

The third article is written by Bethany Gentleman. She provides an overview of the focused subjective and objective assessment of the older adult for critical care nurses. Emphasis is placed on the use of relevant evidence-based screening tools, which may be useful in the care of a critically ill older adult. The fourth article is on ethnogeriatrics and was written after the author, Sonya R. Hardin, completed the Ethnogeriatric Faculty Development Program held yearly at Stanford University in Palo Alto, California. An increase in diversity of older adults is expected to emerge over the next ten years.

Crit Care Nurs Clin N Am 26 (2014) xi–xiii
http://dx.doi.org/10.1016/j.ccell.2013.10.010
0899-5885/14/$ – see front matter © 2014 Elsevier Inc. All rights reserved.

An ethnogeriatric assessment should be included on all admissions to the ICU. This assessment would include information on ethnicity, level of acculturation, religion/spirituality, preferred interaction pattern, facilitation of communication, and any physical examination constraints due to ethnicity.

The fifth article is by Rose Ann DiMaria-Ghalili and Michele Nicolo. It is known that nutrition and hydration are vital components of critical care nursing. However, meeting the nutrition and hydration needs of the critically ill older adult is often complex due to preexisting risk factors (malnutrition, unintentional weight loss, frailty, and dehydration), as well as ICU-related challenges (catabolism, eating and feeding, end-of-life care). This article highlights the challenges of managing nutrition and hydration, reviews assessment principles, and offers strategies for optimizing nutrition and hydration for the critically ill older adult.

The sixth article is on infection, sepsis, and immune function in the critically ill older adult. Written by Camille Lineberry and Deborah E. Stein, the article discusses the vulnerability of older adults and the associated risk of developing sepsis due to functional and immune changes, as well as frequent instrumentation and contact with the health care system. The challenge of recognizing the early signs of sepsis is complicated often by nonspecific complaints. This article addresses how advanced age is an independent predictor of mortality in the septic population of elderly.

The seventh article is focused on cardiovascular issues seen among older adults. Leslie L. Davis discusses select cardiovascular conditions and physiological changes that predispose elders to these conditions; typical signs and symptoms, common diagnostic tests, and evidence-based treatment for this population are included. The implications for nursing care of critically ill elders who have these conditions are also discussed.

The eighth article is written by Delia E. Fredrick on the subject of pulmonary issues in critically ill older adults. Older adults have anatomic and physiologic changes of the protective mechanisms of the pulmonary system that can impact outcomes. She reviews many of the pulmonary changes, such as altered rate and effort of breathing, decreased expiratory strength effort, and impaired oxygenation, that can result in a cognitive change. A number of bedside nursing interventions are discussed, which help to improve patient outcomes.

The ninth article is on renal issues in older adults. Bryan Boling reviews the most commonly encountered complications in the ICU associated with an alteration in kidney function. This article describes the classification of renal dysfunction, the effects of aging on kidney function, as well as additional risk factors, management strategies, and outcomes in the older adult population.

One of the most important systems to ensure a quicker recovery when admitted to an ICU is in the area of mobility. Helen W. Lach, Rebecca A. Lorenz, and Kristine M. L'Ecuyer wrote the tenth article on aging muscles and joints. Critical illness can impose immobility, resulting in loss of strength and functional ability in older patients. The authors discuss how early mobilization programs reduce the impact of immobility and improve outcomes for older patients. The components of a successful mobility program include a good patient assessment, a core set of interventions, and use of the whole health care team.

The eleventh article, on psychiatric disorders, was written by Laura M. Struble, Barbara J. Sullivan, and Laurie S. Hartman. Approximately 30% to 50% of older patients who are hospitalized for a medical condition also have a psychiatric disorder. The intent of this article is to prepare acute care nurses to meet the mental health needs of older adults with critical illness and prevent untoward sequelae of medical events. They discuss the importance of baseline assessment data and manifestations of common psychiatric disorders.

"Delirium in the Older Adult in Critical Care," written by Katheryne Tifuh Amba, is the twelfth article in this issue. The article focuses on the common neurological condition of delirium and how often the challenge exists in diagnosis.

The thirteenth article is written by Roberta Kaplow on the topic of oncologic issues in the older adult. This article describes the pathophysiologic changes that occur with aging as they relate to cancer and cytotoxic therapies, implications for drug therapy, and complications of treatment modalities as they relate to the older person with cancer who may potentially be admitted to the ICU. Knowledge of these issues is essential for health care providers so they can face the complexities that may occur and optimize the outcomes of critically ill older persons diagnosed with cancer.

The fourteenth, and last article in this issue, is on palliative care in the critical care unit. Author Joan E. Dacher discusses the need for palliation, the leadership roles nurses must assume, and barriers to palliative care programs. Her key message is that unless patients and families are offered a choice in care trajectory, many will continue to expect the traditional practice of care. End-of-life discussions are ethically necessary to ensure comfort is provided versus futile care.

I want to personally thank all of the authors of this issue who worked tirelessly to produce information that is important to the care of older adults and critical to the optimal outcomes. Critical care nurses strive to provide safe care and to continually enhance knowledge in the care of patients. I appreciate all the caring moments nurses provide to help the families of older adults at the end of life.

Sonya R. Hardin, PhD, RN, CCRN, NP-C
College of Nursing
East Carolina University
600 Moye Boulevard
Greenville, NC 27858, USA

E-mail address:
srhardin7970@gmail.com

The Epidemiology of Acute and Critical Illness in Older Adults

Linda Bell, RN, MSN

KEYWORDS

- Older adult • Critical care • Acute • Mortality • Transitions

KEY POINTS

- The general population of those over age 65 is increasing as well as that of those over age 85.
- Admissions to medical ICUs increase with aging whereas admissions to surgical ICUs are more likely from procedural complications or trauma.
- Among Medicare patient readmissions, 60% are considered potentially preventable.
- Age over 75 is an independent predictor of mortality in ICU admissions, especially in patients who receive mechanical ventilation.

INTRODUCTION

The population continues to grow across the globe. In 2010, the United Nations estimated the world population at 6.9 billion, with approximately 3.5 billion male and 3.4 billion female. At that time, the estimate for people over age 65 worldwide was approximately 500 million, with 353,000 over age 100.[1] At the same time, population in the United States was more than 300 million. An estimated 43 million of those were over age 65; almost 6 million were over age 85.[2] The 2010 census also found that, for the first time, the number of those aging was increasing rapidly with a concomitant decreasing birth rate.[3] The same census also found that the number of individuals over age 65 living in family households in the United States was twice that of those not living with family; and twice as many women were living alone as were men.[4]

Hospital admissions for individuals over age 65 are measured by admissions from the community and from nursing homes. Community admissions in 2009 were more frequent, at a rate of 310.7/1000 whereas admissions from nursing homes were at a rate of 204.5/1000. Patients admitted from nursing homes had a longer length of stay, however, and were more likely to die in the hospital. Infections, such as septicemia and urinary tract infection (UTI), were the predominant reason for admission from nursing homes. Admission rates for patients over age 65, whether

The author has nothing to disclose.
Technology-Based Learning, American Association of Critical Care Nurses, 101 Columbia, Aliso Viejo, CA 92656, USA
E-mail address: Linda.bell@aacn.org

from community or nursing homes, are at an approximately 2 to 3 times greater rate than for patients under age 65.[5]

ADMISSIONS TO THE ICU

The Society of Critical Care Medicine has estimated approximately 5 million admissions to ICUs per year.[6] Patients over age 65 accounted for 45% of admissions in one study, with 10% of admissions for patients 85 years or older. The percentage of patients admitted to medical ICUs increases per decade after age 65 whereas the percentage of admissions to the surgical intensive care decreases by decade. Trauma and infectious disease admissions increase with advancing age.[7] Patients over 85 are more likely to be admitted to the ICU after a surgical procedure. Patients admitted without an ICU stay had lower inpatient and 90-day mortality for surgical rather than medical admissions.[8]

Primary admitting diagnosis to the ICU in the over-65 age group changes based on the decade. In the 75 to 84 age group, the principal diagnoses in order of frequency are congestive heart failure (CHF), pneumonia, irregular heartbeat, septicemia, osteoarthritis, and chronic obstructive pulmonary disease. In patients over 85 years, the order of frequency changes to CHF, pneumonia, septicemia, UTIs, irregular heartbeat, and hip fractures. The most common procedure for all patients above age 75 is blood transfusion. Procedures for degenerative bone and joint disorders are more common above age 85, with hospitalization for hip fracture 10 times more frequent than for the 75 to 84–year old age group. The most common procedures in hospitalized patients ages 75 to 84 after blood transfusion are diagnostic cardiac procedures, upper gastrointestinal (GI) endoscopy, and respiratory intubation and mechanical ventilation, followed by echocardiogram and hemodialysis. In the 85+-year-old age group, blood transfusions were followed by upper GI endoscopy, respiratory intubation and mechanical ventilation, diagnostic cardiac catheterization, treatment of fracture of dislocation of the hip and femur, and colonoscopy and biopsy.[9,10]

EFFECTS OF AGING AND QUALITY OF LIFE

The US Burden of Disease Collaborators found in reviewing their data on disability-adjusted life years (DALY), healthy life expectancy (HALE), and years lived with disability (YLD) that, although cardiovascular diseases, cancer, and chronic respiratory disease all contribute to YLD, by far the largest contributors are mental/behavioral disorders, such as major depressive disorders, and musculoskeletal disorders, such as low back pain. Although life span is increasing, there is not a decrease in years lived with disability; rather, YLDs increased because onset of disability years has remained stable. Contributors to DALYs were diet, tobacco smoking, high body mass index, high blood pressure, high fasting plasma glucose, physical inactivity, and alcohol use.[11] Gill and colleagues[12] found, however, that the trajectory of disability in their study population was not linked to the cause of death except in the patients with advanced dementia. The goal of Healthy People 2010 was to increase perceived health-related quality of life for both physical and mental health. Key surveillance findings were that the biggest increase in overall unhealthy days occurred between ages 45 and 64; however, although the physically unhealthy days increased in the 65 to 74–year old group mentally, unhealthy days and activity limitation days showed no consistent trends.[13]

Older adults have a higher risk of admission to the ICU secondary to trauma and this risk factor increases with age, most likely due to instability, medications, or strange environments.[7] Scheetz[14] also identified calcium loss with decreased bone density, diminished vision, and cognitive decline as risk factors for injury. The metabolic response to injury is also affected in the older population who may have a decreased sensitivity to intrinsic catecholamine release with subsequent decrease in cardiovascular stimulation. Preinjury malnutrition affects transition from the catabolic to anabolic phase. Wound healing is affected by thinning of the skin and decreased collagen synthesis with an increased risk of infection secondary to changes in immune response related to aging. Delirium and dementia occur at a rate of 8.1 stays/1000 population, which is 7 times the admission rate for 65 to 74 year olds.[9]

TRANSITIONS AND READMISSIONS

Older adult patients with ICU admissions related to trauma/falls are more likely to be discharged to long-term care than patients in the same age group admitted for other diagnoses.[15] Patients age 85 and older are hospitalized at a rate twice that of 65 to 74 year olds and represent a larger share of discharges than their equivalent representation in the total population (8.0/1.8) compared with the 65 to 74–year old group (13.8/4.3% of population). They are also 2.5 times more likely to be discharge to long-term care facilities than the 65 to 74–year old group and have a slightly longer inpatient stay (5.6 compared with 5.3 days).[9]

Data from 2008 showed that 60% of all hospitalizations considered potentially preventable were in patients 65 or older. Although men were more likely to be admitted for potentially preventable conditions, women were more likely to be admitted for preventable acute conditions. Potentially preventable chronic care admissions accounted for 10.1% of Medicare stays whereas 6.8% of stays were attributed to preventable acute care conditions.[16] Krumholtz and colleagues[17] found that strong predictors of mortality were not necessarily strong predictors of readmissions. Patients admitted from the community but discharged to nursing homes were admitted with one of the following: an injury, infection, musculoskeletal disorders, or stroke or other cerebrovascular disease.[7] Also of significance, patients with low health literacy are sicker than a matched group with higher health literacy.[18]

The report of a Robert Wood Johnson Foundation–funded analysis found many themes during interviews with recently discharged patients and families/caregivers. In some cases, patients did not see readmission as a problem, whereas others thought they were discharged too soon without understanding their discharge instructions or that care instructions were not specific enough. Patients found managing new diagnoses challenging; however, those with long-term chronic conditions did not have adequate education about their illness over multiple admissions.[19]

MORTALITY IN HOSPITALIZED OLDER ADULTS

In patients over 75 years, age has been identified as an independent risk factor during ICU admission and the risk continues beyond discharge from the ICU. Risk of death is more likely within 6 months of discharge and among those who received mechanical ventilation.[7] Death rates from complications of both medical and surgical care have been steadily decreasing for all age groups, including those over age 65.[20]

A study in the Netherlands found that poor prognosis and preadmission health status are better predictors of poor outcomes than age alone. This study concluded that the predictive tools currently used to assess prognosis do not adequately evaluate factors affecting older adult patients.[21] This same group developed a model based on the Simplified Acute Physiology Score II model to predict in-hospital mortality for patients 80 years and older.[22]

Data from the National Vital Statistics System for 2012 found that age-adjusted death rates were higher for men than for women for heart disease, cancer, chronic lower respiratory diseases, diabetes, and unintentional injuries. Death from stroke had a similar rate for men and women whereas women had a higher death rate from Alzheimer disease.[23]

Care delivery has been for both aggressive and nonaggressive interventions at the end-of-life, with an increase in the intensity of care. Hospice payments also increased over the period of time studied (1978–2006), however, supporting the authors' conclusion that palliative and supportive care is becoming more common.[24] The national trend in ICU admissions for chronically ill patients at the end of life has been stable from 2007 to 2010 at 3.8 to 3.9 ICU days per patient.[25] From the time period 2000 to 2009, the percentage of Medicare beneficiaries who have ICU admission in the last month of life has increased from 24% in 2000 to 29% in 2009. Health care transitions in the last 3 days of life have increased from 10.3% in 2000 to 14.2% in 2009; 70% of these transitions have been to hospice, whereas only 10% have been to acute care.[26]

SUMMARY

There are several takeaway points from these data. Aging and disease are not synonymous; however, changes related to aging present challenges to those caring for older adults in acute care. Understanding the burden of chronic health conditions in contributing to morbidity and mortality may help in developing educational tools that address the issue of health literacy and promote self-care. Developing appropriate prognostic tools that address age-related changes can help in decision making. Early conversations about end-of-life preferences by primary care practitioners and/ or medical homes can help address issues that arise when older adults are admitted to acute care facilities and provide direction to caregivers in determining care transitions at the end of life.

REFERENCES

1. United Nations Department of Economic and Social Affairs. World population prospects: 2012 revision. Available at: http://esa.un.org/unpd/wpp/Excel-Data/population.htm. Accessed June 18, 2013.
2. United States Census Bureau. Annual estimates of the resident population for selected age groups by sex for the United States, States, Counties, and Puerto Rico Commonwealth and Municipios: April 1, 2010 to July 1, 2012. Available at: http://factfinder2.census.gov/faces/tableservices/jsf/pages/productview.xhtml?pid=PEP_2012_PEPAGESEX&prodType=table. Accessed June 18, 2013.
3. Population Reference Bureau. 2012 World Population Data Set. Available at: http://www.prb.org/pdf12/2012-population-data-sheet_eng.pdf. Accessed June 18, 2013.
4. United States Census Bureau. Population Age 65 Years and Older in the United States. Available at: http://factfinder2.census.gov/faces/tableservices/jsf/pages/productview.xhtml?fpt=table. Accessed June 18, 2003.
5. Spector W, Mutter R, Owens P, et al. Transitions between nursing homes and hospitals in the elderly population 2009. Healthcare Cost and Utilization Project Statistical Brief #141. Rockville (MD): U. S. Agency for Healthcare Research and Quality; 2012.
6. Society of Critical Care Medicine. Critical Care Statistics. Available at: http://www.sccm.org/Communications/Pages/CriticalCareStats.aspx. Accessed July 1, 2013.

7. Fuchs L, Chronaki CE, Park S, et al. ICU admission characteristics and mortality rates among elderly and very elderly patients. Intensive Care Med 2012;38: 1654–61.
8. Yu W, Ash AS, Levinsky NG, et al. Intensive care unit use and mortality in the elderly. J Gen Intern Med 2000;15:97–102.
9. Weir L, Pfuntner A, Steiner C. Hospital utilization among the oldest adults, 2008. Healthcare Cost and utilization Project Statistical brief #103. Rockville (MD): Agency for Healthcare Research and Quality; 2010.
10. Joynt KE, Gawande AA, Orav EJ, et al. Contribution of preventable acute care spending to total spending for high-cost medicare patients. JAMA 2013; 309(24):2572–8.
11. Murray CJL, Abraham J, Ali MK, et al. The state of US health, 1990-2010: burden of diseases, injuries, and risk factors. JAMA 2013;310(6):591–608.
12. Gill TM, Gahbauer EA, Han L, et al. Trajectories of disability in the last year of life. N Engl J Med 2010;362:1173–80.
13. Moriarty DG, Kobau R, Zack MM, et al. Tracking healthy days - a window on the health of older adults. Prev Chronic Dis 2005;2(3):A16. Available at: http://www.cdc.gov/pcd/issues/205/jul/05_0023htm.
14. Scheetz LJ. Life-threatening injuries in older adults. AACN Adv Crit Care 2011; 22(2):128–39.
15. Grimm D, Mion LC. Falls resulting in traumatic injury among older adults. AACN Adv Crit Care 2011;22(2):161–9.
16. Stranges E, Stocks C. Potentially preventable hospitalizations for acute and chronic conditions, 2008. Healthcare cost and utilization project statistical brief #99. Rockville (MD): Agency for Healthcare Research and Utilization; 2010.
17. Krumholtz H, Lin A, Keenan PS, et al. Relationship between hospital readmission and mortality rates for patients hospitalized with acute myocardial infarction, heart failure, or pneumonia. JAMA 2013;309(6):587–93.
18. Cloonan P, Wood J, Riley JB. Reducing 30-day readmissions. J Nurs Adm 2013; 43(7–8):382–7.
19. Perry M. Hospital readmissions from the inside out: stories from patients and health care providers. In: The revolving door: a report on U. S. hospital readmissions. Princeton, NJ: Robert Wood Johnson Foundation; 2013. p. 32–56.
20. Centers for Disease Control and Prevention. QuickStats: death rate from complications of medical and surgical care among adults aged >45 years, by age group – United States, 1999-2009. MMWR Morb Mortal Wkly Rep 2012;61(37):750.
21. Rooij SE, Abu-Hanna A, Levi M, et al. Factors that predict outcome of intensive care treatment in very elderly patients: a review. Crit Care 2005;9:R307–14.
22. Rooij SE, Abu-Hanna A, Levi M, et al. Identification of high-risk subgroups in very elderly intensive care unit patients. Crit Care 2007;11:R33.
23. US Department of Health and Human Services. Health, United States, 2012 with Special Feature on Emergency Care. Table 20. Available at: http://www.cdc.gov/nchs/data/hus/hus12.pdf. Accessed July 4, 2013.
24. Riley GF, Lubitz JD. Long-term trends in medicare payments in the last year of life. Health Serv Res 2010;45(2):565–76.
25. Goodman DC, Fisher ED, Wennberg JE, et al. Tracking improvement in the care of chronically ill patients: a dartmouth atlas brief on medicare beneficiaries near the end-of-life. Hanover (NH): A Report of the Dartmouth Atlas Project; 2013.
26. Teno JM, Cozalo PL, Bynum JP, et al. Change in end-of-life care for medicare beneficiaries: site of death, place of care, and health care transitions in 2000, 2005, and 2009. JAMA 2013;309(5):470–7.

The Impact of Aging Physiology in Critical Care

Mandi Walker, MSN, RN-BC, CCRN*, Mark Spivak, BSN, RN, CEN,
Mary Sebastian, MHA, BSN, CNML

KEYWORDS

- Aging • Physiology • Critical care • Geriatric

KEY POINTS

- Managing the aging critically ill patient is highly complex and necessitates a comprehensive understanding of the normal physiologic changes that occur with aging.
- Age alone should not be considered a primary factor in the prognosis of critically ill patients.
- The practitioner must take comorbidities and functional disabilities into account, along with quality of life and the likelihood of recovery when determining care modalities in the geriatric population.
- All factors regarding the aging patient's plan of care, prognosis, and predicted quality of life should be openly and honestly discussed with patients and/or their families to ensure all decisions regarding care are fully informed.
- Future research surrounding the care of the older critically ill patient should include a comprehensive study of the impact of aging on diagnosis and treatment modalities that impact the underlying mechanisms of aging.
- Additional studies focusing specifically on the effects of aging and the critically ill patient are needed to add to this body of knowledge.
- In particular, the incorporation of evidence-based practice and nurse-driven protocols may have a positive impact on the care and outcome of these patients.

INTRODUCTION

The US population is aging at a rate faster than ever before.[1] The elderly represent a significant proportion of patients seeking care, who present more acute, get admitted more frequently, and account for as much as 50% of all intensive care unit admissions, and this number is only projected to grow.[1–4] These patients are at greater risk for complications during their admission, extended lengths of stay, and becoming chronically ill following their hospitalization.[1]

Nursing Education and Research Department, University of Louisville Hospital, 530 South Jackson Street, Louisville, KY 40202, USA
* Corresponding author.
E-mail address: mandiwa@ulh.org

Crit Care Nurs Clin N Am 26 (2014) 7–14
http://dx.doi.org/10.1016/j.ccell.2013.09.005
0899-5885/14/$ – see front matter © 2014 Elsevier Inc. All rights reserved.

ccnursing.theclinics.com

The words of Justice Potter Stewart[5] "I don't know what it is, but I know it when I see it," can easily be applied to the definition of old. Scholars vary in their opinion of what defines old, but generally it is agreed that 65 and older is considered to be old age. Aging can be further subcategorized as young old (65–74), middle old (75–84) and old old (85+).[4] Regardless of how one categorizes age, it is recognized that significant changes in physiology related to the aging process are present in varying degrees by the age of 65.[1–4]

Aging does not accelerate over the life span; however, age-related changes have a greater accumulation in an older patient versus a middle-aged patient.[6] Progressive deterioration, which begins as subtle changes early on, continues throughout the aging process. The rate of change varies between individuals and among organ systems.[1] Factors contributing to the extent of aging physiology in elderly patients include genetics, lifestyle, and environment.[2] The impact of aging physiology in critical care is further compounded by the presence of comorbidities, which are more prevalent in the aging population.[3,7] Therefore, chronologic and biologic ages do not parallel one another, making the aging process patient specific, and the care of these patients of necessity individualized.[1,8]

An aging patient will not be able to mount the same hemodynamic and metabolic response to the stress of a critical illness as a younger patient.[7] This lack of resilience may lead to atypical presentation of severe illness, and may lead to delays in diagnosis and treatment.[9] For instance, an aging patient presenting with neurologic compromise, such as confusion, dizziness, and decreased level of consciousness, may not necessarily indicate a neurologic issue, but instead may mask infection, electrolyte imbalances, cardiac dysfunction, or drug toxicity, causing a delay in proper diagnosis.[9]

AGING PHYSIOLOGY
Cellular

Although the effects of aging may be visible at a macro level while observing a patient in the critical care unit, the true impact of what is occurring needs to be understood at the micro level. Changes at the cellular level impact all physiologic processes. Given that the effects of aging are mostly observed superficially, they begin and are at play on the cellular level well before being visualized. Before the first wrinkle is noted on a forehead or at the corner of the eyes, free radicals are bombarding cells from both within and outside the cell membrane, disrupting their ability to carry on with normal activity, communicate with other cells, and propagate new cells to take their place.[10,11]

Aging cells display a greater amount of damage compared with their younger counterparts.[10] An increase in cellular superoxide could be a significant factor in the ability of a cell to function.[2,10] In addition, certain enzymes have been identified to have protective properties for the mitochondrial wall of aging cells, and can slow the effects of aging in these cells.[10] Conversely, the lack of these enzymes in laboratory mice showed substantial acceleration in age and loss of skeletal muscle.[10] Wu and colleagues[11] provided evidence regarding mechanotransduction in the aging cell. The process of cellular mechanotransduction is defined as, "the ability of the cell to sense, process, and respond to mechanical stimuli and is an important regulator of physiologic function that has been found to play a role in regulating gene expression, protein synthesis, cell differentiation, tissue growth, and most recently, the pathophysiology of disease."[11(p1)] It is believed that with age the ability of the cells to correctly mechanotransduce information becomes damaged, or limited.[10]

Neurologic

It is a misconception that intelligence declines with age. It does not. Brain size and cerebral perfusion decrease with age[7]; this is paralleled with a decrease in functional neurons, resulting in diminished motor function, hearing, vision, and memory.[3,7,12] These changes, along with a prevalence of dementia anywhere from 10% to 18% in persons over 65 years,[13] contribute greatly to the care required of critically ill older adults.[7] Changes in anatomy, along with a decline in cognitive function can complicate neurologic examinations, masking symptoms of acute neurologic disease processes.[3,12] For instance, the decrease in brain size coupled with the greater adherence of the dura to the skull causes a stretching of the bridging vessels in the brain, thereby making an epidural bleed less likely while tripling the possibility of a subdural hematoma in even minor head traumas.[4,12] The increase in dead space also delays onset of symptoms, making close monitoring and careful assessment of an aging patient's neurologic function critical.[3,12]

Although maintaining adequate cerebral perfusion pressure in any critically ill patient is important, a pre-existing decrease in cerebral perfusion predisposes geriatric patients to concomitant neurologic insult, even in non-neurological conditions.[3,7,13] More so in the older adult, the practitioner should pay particular attention to maintaining adequate oxygenation and perfusion throughout the hospitalization. Additionally, it has been shown that the presence or absence of cognitive decline during a critical illness is a predictive factor in the elderly patient's ability to recover and quality of life.[7,13]

Cardiovascular

Many structural changes in the heart and vasculature occur as a natural part of the aging process. This is compounded by the fact that age is a major risk factor in the development of cardiovascular disease.[1,2] Cardiovascular disease alone accounts for greater than 40% of deaths in patients older than 65 years.[1,2,8,13] A lack of cardiac reserve is also noted in most patients by the age of 70.[1–3,7,13]

Significant cardiac structural changes with age include increased interstitial fibrosis of the myocardium, resulting in stiffness and thickening of the cardiac muscle.[1,2,8] Connective tissue and fat replace autonomic tissue, resulting in conduction abnormalities, making dysrhythmias such as sick sinus syndrome, atrial dysrhythmias, atrioventricular blocks, and bundle branch blocks more likely.[1,2,7,12,13] Additionally, up to 78% of patients over the age of 70 have significant amyloid deposits within the myocardium, further contributing to the stiffening of the muscle wall and increasing the likelihood of these conduction defects and subsequent heart failure.[1,6]

Systolic blood pressure significantly rises with age, while diastolic blood pressure rises to a lesser extent, leading to an increase in pulse pressure.[7,8,12] Cardiac output decreases in an aging heart, putting the elderly patient at a disadvantage when faced with increased metabolic demand.[1,2,6,7,12,13] Although basal heart rate remains relatively unchanged with age, the aging heart is less susceptible to sympathetic stimulation, so it cannot compensate for an increased need of cardiac output by significantly increasing the heart rate.[1–3,6–8,12,13] Additionally, there is an increased afterload caused by increase in aortic and carotid artery wall thickness and less elasticity in the vasculature.[1–3,6–8,12,13] Instead, the aging heart meets this increased need by increasing ventricular filling and stroke volume, but this also causes more work for the heart, and making it preload-dependent and less adaptable in hypovolemic states.[1,2,7,8,12,13] Maintaining adequate circulating volume is crucial in geriatric patients.[2,3,13] However, this must be balanced with a decrease in ventricular compliance and the risk of over-resuscitating the patient, causing pulmonary edema.[2,13]

Pulmonary

The aging lung is less able to defend itself from the insult of trauma and illness. Chest wall compliance decreases with the development of kyphosis, calcification of the costal cartilage, vertebral collapse, and atrophy of the respiratory muscles.[1,2,8,12–14] These changes make the patient's cough less effective, and decreases the patient's maximal inspiratory and expiratory force by up to 50%, leading to an increased effort of breathing, expending more energy for the same amount of inspiratory work.[1,2,8,12–14] Because of the decrease in air movement within the lung during ventilation, breath sounds will be diminished.[8] Although these are not noticeable in a healthy older person, the impact is significant in the presence of an acute illness.[1]

Lung compliance diminishes with a decrease in elasticity and recoil.[1,8,12,14] This is coupled with the loss of alveolar surface area, surfactant, and ciliary clearance.[1,2,12,13] The result is a higher residual lung volume and air trapping, and a decrease in surface area for gas exchange, leading to ventilation–perfusion (V/Q) mismatches.[1,2,8,12,14] Arterial oxygen tension (PaO_2) decreases approximately 0.3 mmHg/year (milimeters of mercury) after age 30, leading to a normal range of 60 to 80 in the elderly.[1,2,12–14] Conversely, arterial carbon dioxide tension ($PaCO_2$) does not alter with age, so hypercapnia or hypocapnia should be considered pathologic.[1,2,8,12]

Chemoreceptor function and respiratory center functions alter with age, leaving the elderly patient less able to respond to hypoxia and hypercapnia.[1,2,12–14] Vigilance is warranted when assessing and monitoring these patients, as they may not show visible signs of distress.[1,12] These patients have a decreased respiratory reserve, and can decompensate quickly.[1,12,13]

Older adults are at higher risk of developing pneumonia due to the decrease in immunologic functioning and airway clearance.[8,14] Management of a geriatric patient with pneumonia does not vary from that of the younger patient.[8] However, every effort should be made to prevent the development of pneumonia in the aging patient, as the mortality rate for pneumonia within this population is 5 times greater.[8]

Although evidence varies regarding the use of mechanical ventilation in the elderly, studies indicate that age alone should not be a deterrent.[2,8,14] Instead the patient's overall condition, prior smoking history, comorbidities, and disease prognosis should be taken into account.[8,14,15] The development of complications while ventilated is also a contributory factor to the elderly patient's survival, so utilizing care bundles and evidence-based practice to prevent these complications is key to the patient's recovery.[8,9,14] Nappagan and Parker[8] suggest the use of the organ failure system index to predict outcomes with the use of mechanical ventilation. Weaning from the ventilator may be prolonged in the aging patient due to the increase in work of breathing and muscle atrophy during mechanical ventilation.[2,13,14]

Gastrointestinal

Many changes occur within the gastrointestinal (GI) tract and liver during the aging process. A decrease in absorption can lead to underlying nutritional deficits, especially protein deficits.[2,7,12] Therefore, close attention to the patient's nutritional status and early support, with an emphasis on protein, is important to overall outcome in this patient population.[2,7,12]

A decrease in motility, delayed emptying of the stomach, and an increased incidence of diverticula are common in the aging adult. These put the critical care patient at an increased risk for aspiration, as well as constipation, obstruction, ileus, and perforation.[3,6] In addition, there is a decrease in acid secretion and mucous production that weakens the lining of intestinal walls and can lead to bacterial over-growth, putting the gut at risk for acute GI bleeds and bacterial translocation into the systemic circulation.[7]

Renal

Significant changes in the renal system during aging include a decrease in renal size of up to 30% by age 80 and renal blood flow up to 50%.[6,7] This underlying decrease in renal perfusion puts the aging patient at risk for acute renal failure from even minor hy-potensive insults.[1–3,12,13] Between the ages of 25 and 85, about 40% of nephrons become sclerotic.[1,2,13] There is also a decrease in afferent and efferent renal arterioles and renal tubular cell number.[1,2,13] These factors contribute to a diminished capacity to concentrate urine, conserve sodium, and excrete hydrogen, leading to fluid and acid base imbalances.[2,7,8,13] Aging patients are at risk to become dehydrated, which can complicate the previously discussed preload-dependent cardiovascular changes.[7] All of these changes may be related to alterations in the renin–angiotensin system.[1,2]

A decrease in glomerular filtration rate (GFR) of up to 50% can impact the patient's ability to metabolize drugs cleared through the kidneys.[2,7,8,12,13] In some instances, the half-life of renally cleared drugs can double in the presence of renal impairment.[6,12] Despite the reduction in GFR, serum creatinine remains unchanged related to a par-allel decrease in lean body mass, and may not accurately reflect the patient's true renal function.[2,6,7] Conversely, creatinine clearance is affected by the decrease in GFR, up to 33%.[7] Consideration should be given to the use of creatinine clearance for dosage calculation of renally metabolized drugs, as this may be more accurate than basing dosage on serum creatinine alone.[1,2] In addition to creatinine clearance, serum urea nitrogen (BUN) has been recommended as a useful tool to evaluate overall renal function in an elderly patient.[7]

Musculoskeletal

Aging-related changes to the musculoskeletal system begin at age 30.[12] A person loses 3% to 4% of his or her bony mass each decade.[12] Ligaments and joints tend to stiffen ,with resulting loss of flexibility,[12] and cartilage strength decreases.[3] The presence of osteoarthritis and narrowing of the cervical canal place these patients at a high risk for spinal cord damage from even minor trauma.[12]

Most changes in the mobility of elderly patients are related to skeletal alterations, but a decrease in muscle strength is also a contributory factor. By 80 years of age, ad-ipose tissue increases while lean body mass decreases by up to 40%.[2,7,8,12] Cellular mechanotransduction plays a significant role in this process.[11] According to Wu and colleagues[11] the mechanotransduction process becomes damaged in the aging pro-cess, resulting in ineffective regulation of muscle mass throughout the body, leading to muscle atrophy in geriatric patients. Clinical studies indicate age-related loss of mus-cle mass dramatically increases by more than fourfold from ages 70 to 75 to 85 and older.[11]

Age-related musculoskeletal deterioration may be further influenced by hormone changes, malnutrition, and a decrease in activity.[8,13] Overall, the aging process makes geriatric patients more susceptible to fractures, tears, and dislocation from even minor-to-moderate trauma.[3,4,12] The decrease in muscle mass is also found to contribute to the likelihood of patient falls and the ability to recuperate from such falls.[3] This has significant consequences on not only their quality of life, but their ability to care for themselves as aging occurs.

Integumentary

The major changes in the integumentary system during aging include a loss of subcutaneous adipose tissue and atrophy of the epidermis layer of the skin, putting the patient at a greater risk for injury and infection.[3,12] A decrease in epidermal cell growth and division, as well as a decrease in dermal vasculature, can contribute to a higher incidence of decubitus ulcers in the aging patient.[6,12] Loss of skin tone and elasticity

Table 1 System overview		
System	System Changes After 65 Years of Age	Impact of Changes
Cellular	• Impaired cellular communication • Diminished capacity to replicate	• Impacts all body systems at their basic level to function and propagate
Neurologic	• Decreased brain size • Diminished cerebral perfusion • Fewer functional neurons	• Diminished motor function, hearing, vision, and memory • Predictive of recovery and quality of life
Cardiovascular	• Thick, stiff myocardium • Conduction abnormalities • Less responsive to sympathetic stimulation	• Preload-dependent • Susceptible to dysrhythmias • Less adaptable in hypovolemic states
Pulmonary	• Decreased chest wall compliance • Diminished elasticity and recoil • Loss of alveolar surface area, surfactant, and ciliary clearance	• V/Q mismatches • Decreased airway clearance • Risk for developing pneumonia • Prolonged ventilator weaning
GI	• Decrease in absorption • Decreased motility • Delayed gastric emptying • Decreased acid secretion and mucous production • Weakened intestinal wall	• Nutritional deficits, especially protein • Risk for aspiration, constipation, obstruction, ileus, and perforation • Risk for acute GI bleeds and bacterial translocation into the systemic circulation
Renal	• Decreased renal mass and perfusion • Sclerotic nephrons • Decreased number of afferent and efferent renal arterioles and renal tubular cells • Decreased GFR	• Fluid and acid base imbalances • Diminished capacity to concentrate urine, conserve sodium, and excrete hydrogen • Delayed drug metabolism through the kidneys
Musculoskeletal	• Stiffening of ligaments and joints • Decreased muscle & cartilage strength • Presence of osteoarthritis and narrowing of the cervical canal	• Loss of flexibility • Susceptible to fractures, tears, and dislocation • Increased likelihood of falls
Integumentary	• Loss of subcutaneous adipose tissue • Atrophy of the epidermis • Stiffening of the dermal collagen and calcification of elastin	• Greater risk for injury and infection • Higher incidence of decubitus ulcers • Loss of skin tone and elasticity • Prolonged healing

is common in older adults.[6] This is caused by a combination of the stiffening and loss of pliability of the dermal collagen and the calcification of elastin.[6] Injuries to the skin in an older adult may take up to twice as long to re-epithelialize compared with younger adults.[6]

SUMMARY

Managing the aging critically ill patient is highly complex and necessitates a comprehensive understanding of the normal physiologic changes that occur with aging. **Table 1** provides a summary of the physiologic changes that occur with aging. However, age alone should not be considered a primary factor in the prognosis of critically ill patients.[3,7,16] Comorbidities and functional disabilities, which increase with advancing age, further complicate care.[3,7,16] The practitioner must take these into account, along with quality of life and the likelihood of recovery when determining care modalities in the geriatric population.[14] All factors regarding the aging patient's plan of care, prognosis, and predicted quality of life should be openly and honestly discussed with patients and/or their families to ensure all decisions regarding care are fully informed.[14,17]

Future research surrounding the care of the older critically ill patient should include a comprehensive study of the impact of aging on diagnosis and treatment modalities that impact the underlying mechanisms of aging. Available evidence is limited and somewhat outdated. Additional studies focusing specifically on the effects of aging and the critically ill patient are needed to add to this body of knowledge. In particular, the incorporation of evidence-based practice and nurse-driven protocols may have a positive impact on the care and outcome of these patients.[9]

REFERENCES

1. Menaker J, Scalea TM. Geriatric care in the surgical intensive care unit. Crit Care Med 2010;38(9):S452–9.
2. Marik PE. Management of the critically ill geriatric patient. Crit Care Med 2006; 34(9):S176–82.
3. Thompson HJ, Bourbonniere M. Traumatic injury in the older adult from head to toe. Crit Care Nurs Clin N Am 2006;18(3):419–31.
4. Young L, Ahmad H. Trauma in the elderly: a new epidemic? Aust N Z J Surg 1999; 69:584–6.
5. Stewart P, Jacobellis v Ohio, 378 US 184 (1964).
6. Boss GR, Seegmiller JE. Age-related physiological changes and their clinical significance. Geriatric Med West J Med 1981;135:434–40.
7. Mick DJ, Ackerman MH. Critical care nursing for older adults: pathophysiological and functional considerations. Nurs Clin N Am 2004;39:473–93.
8. Nagappan R, Parkin G. Geriatric critical care. Crit Care Clin 2003;19:253–70.
9. Casey CM, Balas MC. Use of protocols in older intensive care unit patients. AACN Advanced Critical Care 2011;22(2):150–60.
10. Jackson MJ. Skeletal muscle aging: role of reactive oxygen species. Crit Care Med 2009;37(10):S368–71.
11. Wu M, Fannin J, Rice KM, et al. Effect of aging on cellular mechanotransduction. Aging Research Reviews 2011;10:1–15.
12. Gillies D. Elderly trauma: they are different. Australian Critical Care 1999; 12(1):24–30.
13. Pisani MA. Considerations in caring for the critically ill older patient. Journal of Intensive Care Medicine 2009;24(2):83–95.

14. Phelan BA, Cooper DA, Sangkachand P. Prolonged mechanical ventilation and tracheostomy in the elderly. AACN Clinical Issues 2002;13(1):84–93.

15. Farfel JM, Franca SA, Sitta Mdo S, et al. Age, invasive ventilator support and outcomes in elderly patients admitted to the intensive care unit. Age and Ageing 2009;38:515–20.

16. Endeman H, Heeffer L, Holleman F, et al. Influence of old age on survival after prolonged mechanical ventilation. European Journal of Internal Medicine 2005; 16:116–9.

17. Institute for Family-Centered Care. 2010. Available at: http://www.ipfcc.org/faq.html. Accessed February 20, 2013.

Focused Assessment in the Care of the Older Adult

Bethany Gentleman, MS, GNP-BC

KEYWORDS

- Focused older adult assessment • Geriatric assessment tools • Critical care

KEY POINTS

- Assessment of the critically ill older adult is focused and based on knowledge of the distinct, defining features of this population.
- Nursing practice is guided by evidence-based methods and is individualized according to the elder's unique health condition and requirements.
- Effective communication is fundamental in acquiring accurate and relevant information about the older adult's history.

INTRODUCTION

The focused assessment approach for the older adult differs markedly to that for the younger adult. Irrespective of the number and severity of diagnoses, the process demands a high degree of detail and greater concentration of time. This approach presents challenges for the critical care nurse in the rapid-paced care setting where economy of time is essential.

While acknowledging that this population is widely heterogeneous, there are common themes that occur when an older adult is afflicted with a change in health status. The interplay of normal aging changes with individual functional abilities and the commonly high prevalence of underlying chronic comorbidities define the complexity of the elder's response to illness. Diminished physiologic reserve attributable to aging and commonly associated lower resilience pose a high risk for complications of both critical illness and hospitalization.

In the setting of critical illness, the older adult characteristically presents atypically and subtly when decompensation occurs. One decompensating system affects another, often resulting in a rapid cascade of deterioration in an older adult. These factors compel that the critical care nurse's assessment skills are astute and have an anticipatory focus.

No disclosures to report.
Private Practice, 9E Gregory Island Road, Hamilton, MA 01982, USA
E-mail address: bethgentleman@verizon.net

Crit Care Nurs Clin N Am 26 (2014) 15–20
http://dx.doi.org/10.1016/j.ccell.2013.09.006
0899-5885/14/$ – see front matter © 2014 Elsevier Inc. All rights reserved.

This article describes the focused subjective and objective assessment of the older adult, with the emphasis on the geriatric specific domains that delineate the assessment of the older from the younger adult. Relevant evidence-based screening tools that the nurse can use in assessing the critically ill older adult are discussed.

FOCUSED ASSESSMENT

A traditional description of the focused assessment highlights the application of skills appropriate to the urgency and pertinence of the primary concern, typically confined to the body system.[1] For the critically ill older adult, the assessment must be collective yet focused. While acuity of the assessment is prioritized to the disease-specific organ system, nursing assessment must consider the elder in the context of the whole person and the environment, and their interactions. Assessment of older adults also integrates a focus on function. The idiom of function relative to the older adult broadly comprises the physical, cognitive, psychological, and social domains.[2] An appraisal of actual or potential geriatric-specific problems within the functional domains will aid in identification of risk for decompensation. Deficiencies and deteriorations, whether singular or in combination, raise the risk for poor outcomes.

A framework for nursing assessment and care pertinent to the older adult is presented in The American Nurse Association (ANA) *Scope and Standards of Practice for Geron-tological Nursing*.[3] The ANA acknowledges the unique defining characteristics of the aging process and specific domains in the care of the older adult, which are outlined as the physiologic, developmental, psychological, economic, cultural, and spiritual.

The standards are intended to reflect the priorities of gerontological nursing, and are a model for care across settings, including critical care. The first of the 6 Standards of Practice, Assessment, includes authoritative statements outlining the expectations for the distinct actions that nurses should competently perform. The Assessment Standard captures the unique considerations of the older adult for nurses to include in the assessment.[3]

Nursing practice is guided by evidence-based methods, and is individualized according to the elder's unique health condition and requirements. The focused assessment of the critically ill elder is divided into 2 components: assessment of preadmission baseline information and ongoing individualized assessment.[4] Establishing a baseline of information allows for comparison in gauging changes, identification of risks, and uncovering signs of complications. This information then guides the planning of care for the individual. Baseline assessment data are gathered within the domains as described earlier.[2,3] Ongoing individualized assessment is aimed at identification of change from baseline, whether deleterious or improved, and from within organ systems and the geriatric-specific domains, for appraisal of new superimposed illness and complications.

Many assessment tools are available for use by the nurse to obtain baseline data, monitor trends that indicate change in condition, and monitor response to plans of care. The Hartford Institute of Geriatric Nursing of New York University, College of Nursing, has produced the *"Try This" Assessment Series*. This compilation of geriatric assessment tools, each with a description of its use, can be accessed directly from the care unit at http://consultgerirn.org.[5] Several of the tools in the series, which are relevant to specific domains of the focused assessment of older adults, are referred to throughout the remainder of this article. Individual variations in level of consciousness and severity of illness will predict the suitability of using the assessment tool at any given time.

BASELINE ASSESSMENT

Effective communication is fundamental in acquiring accurate and relevant information about the older adult's history, goals, and perceptions of and response to the current illness. The presence of serious or life-threatening illness as well as sensory, technological, or cognitive restrictions imposes limitations to procuring necessary baseline and ongoing information. If the elder is incapable of providing self-reported baseline information, family members or significant others are a valuable and recommended source to enlist. Working with families of hospitalized older adults with dementia[6] is a useful tool that can be used to obtaining necessary baseline information from a family member or significant other. The 20-question form addresses information about activities of daily living, falls, behavior, language, and speech, among other baseline information.

Baseline assessment should begin with knowledge of the older adult's medical, psychiatric, surgical, and vaccination history. Inquire also about alcohol, tobacco, and illicit drug use, past or present.[4] Ask for a description of a usual day, elimination patterns, and sleep routines and quality of sleep. The nurse should then inquire about baseline status among the geriatric function-focused domains (physical, cognitive, psychological, and social). Be certain to ask about known visual or hearing deficits and the use of eyeglasses or hearing aids.

Information about the older adult's preadmission cognitive status guides in an understanding of decisional capacity, and in recognizing an underlying impairment that may otherwise go undetected. Elders with preexisting cognitive impairment are at greater risk for development of geriatric syndromes such as delirium,[7] and a change from baseline cognition could signal its evolution. The nurse should inquire about observed problems with memory or episodes of confusion.

Inquiry about changes in interests, mood, and affect may also uncover symptoms of preadmission depression. The elder capable of responding may be asked directly if he or she often feels sad or depressed. An affirmative response would then direct the nurse to expand on the assessment with a standardized instrument. The Geriatric Depression Scale (GDS) is a 15-item scored "yes/no" questionnaire that assesses depression symptoms. This tool has been cited for its usefulness in the acute setting.[8]

Asking about the older adult's ability to perform tasks such as managing the checkbook and finances, medications, and planning and preparing meals reveals details of baseline executive functioning relative to cognitive function. Additional inquiry about how food is obtained and the average daily dietary intake provides a valuable indication of the elder's nutritional status and of existing or anticipated problems. The nurse should also inquire about the older adult's communication abilities, typical interaction patterns, and usual response to stimuli. Knowledge of all medications taken before admission will alert the nurse to the potential for withdrawal issues.[4]

Psychosocial assessment includes baseline information about the elder's marital status, sources of support, family relationships and responsibilities, home and financial situation, religious affiliation, and spirituality. Ask what primary language is spoken, and about cultural values and health beliefs. Impaired baseline abilities to perform the activities of daily living (ADLs) has been associated with poor outcomes, and a decline from baseline can result as a complication of, or herald the onset of a superimposed acute illness. It is vital to inquire about baseline abilities and level of assistance necessary in the ADLs, which include bathing, dressing, feeding, toileting, transferring, and continence. The Katz Index of Independence in Activities of Daily Living tool (Katz ADL) measures the ability of the older adult to perform each of the ADLs, and is scored based on level of ability or impairment.[9] Assessment should also include inquiry about the use of assistive devices, a history of recent falls, and the presence of chronic pain.

Assessment of elder mistreatment among hospitalized older adults has been recommended by the American Medical Association.[10] Screening tools currently available depend on input from the cognitively intact elder or the clinician's observations, and 2 tools screen the caregiver.[11] Although current screening of a family member's or significant other's observations is lacking, information gathered in the previously mentioned cognitive, psychosocial, and functional domains may uncover risk factors inherent to mistreatment.[10]

Knowledge of the older adult's advance directives, wishes, and information relative to a surrogate decision maker is vital. Gaining an understanding of the older adult's goals, values, and hopes is critical in aiding the planning for care appropriate to individual wishes.

The focused physical assessment of the older adult is organized to include the general overview, and assessment from within the perspectives of the geriatric domains and the organ systems. Assessment techniques of each of the organ systems, prioritized and directed by the elder's admitting diagnoses, parallel those for the younger adult.

The general overview, similar to the assessment for the younger adult, encompasses the patient's appearance and the immediate environment. Observe the elder's skin color for a cyanotic, pink, or pallid appearance, level of consciousness, respiratory pattern, and involuntary movements as indicators of distress. Observe for the presence and number of attachments to the elder, such as central lines, intravenous and indwelling bladder catheters, monitoring equipment, and endotracheal intubation.

Assess the oral cavity for the condition of the membranes, gums, teeth, and tongue. Accumulated oral bacteria due to dental caries and periodontal disease have been associated with a high risk for systemic diseases, including aspiration pneumonia.[12] The Kayser-Jones Brief Oral Health Assessment Examination (BOHSE) is a useful screening tool for use by nurses.[13] In the immediate patient environment, note the level of lighting and noise.

Vision and hearing assessment is paramount because sensory deficits have been associated with risks for falls and delirium.[14] The elder's ability to interact with clinicians and family members, and to perceive and comprehend environmental cues, depends on adequate visual and auditory function. A rapid assessment of vision can be accomplished by asking the older adult to read available print on paper. If the elder is not easily responding to conversation, hearing can be assessed by whispering 2 words into each ear from a distance of 1 to 2 feet from the ear. This action may require raising the whisper, then using voice tone until the sound is recognized.[1]

Assessment of cognition can be accomplished by simply talking with the elder who is conscious and able to communicate. Ask an open-ended question to address attention, or ask the elder to recite the months in the year backward. To rapidly assess recall, ask the elder to recall 3 words after 1 minute of hearing and repeating them.[2] The brief established instrument, the Mini-Cog, provides an objective measure of registration, recall, and executive function. The tool is composed of a 3-item recall and the Clock Drawing Test (CDT)[15]; however, for the latter portion the elder must be able to hold a pencil and write.

Early detection of delirium, a common geriatric syndrome associated with poor outcomes in acutely ill hospitalized older adults, can be achieved by using the Confusion Assessment Method for the Intensive Care Unit (CAM-ICU) instrument.

The CAM-ICU was developed to measure delirium risk specifically among critically ill nonverbal patients in the ICU setting, and its usefulness by bedside nurses has been demonstrated.[16]

Continuous assessment of medications for adverse drug events (ADE) is imperative. Older adults are typically on a higher number of medications than are younger adults. In addition to normal pharmacokinetic and pharmacodynamic changes with aging, this places the older adult at high risk for iatrogenesis, drug-to-drug interactions, and ADE,[17] potentially affecting all systems. The Beers Criteria[18] is an evidence-based, informative resource outlining high-risk medications for this population which, if they must be used, can raise the nurse's awareness of the potential for ADE, thereby warranting closer monitoring.

Immobility as a result of serious illness and hospitalization requires that the nurse assess the capacity of physical function systematically and regularly. The previously cited Katz ADL tool also serves as an objective measure of the elder's abilities in the ADL functional measures. This tool can augment the nursing assessment of the elder's musculature for evidence of muscle wasting, level of strength, and range of motion. Carefully observe for signs of pain at rest and with movement.

The elder who has suffered mistreatment may have been admitted as a result of the sequelae of abuse or neglect. Stigmata to be mindful of in the assessment include an unexplained injury, malnutrition, or dehydration.[2] The Elder Assessment Instrument (EAI) is a screening tool for use by a designated clinician if mistreatment is suspected. Though not a scoring tool, recommendations for a social services referral are defined.[19]

SUMMARY

The critical care nurse encounters the highest level of exacting clinical circumstances. The many challenges of assessment and care of the critically ill older adult rely on nursing skills that are focused, discerning, and based on knowledge of the distinct, defining features of this population. Utilization of applicable assessment tools can efficiently support appraisal of stability or change within the domains unique to this population.

REFERENCES

1. Bickley LS, Szilagyi PG, editors. Bates' guide to physical examination and history taking. New York: Wolters Kluwer; Lippincott Williams & Wilkins; 2009. p. 4–5, 226.
2. Flaherty E, Resnick B, editors. Geriatric nursing review syllabus: a core curriculum in advanced practice geriatric nursing. 3rd edition. New York: American Geriatrics Society; 2011. p. 43–4, 88.
3. American Nurses Association. Gerontological nursing: scope and standards of practice. 3rd edition. Silver Spring (MD): Nursesbooks.org; 2010. p. 29.
4. Balas MC, Casey CM, Happ MB. Critical care comprehensive assessment and management of the critically ill. In: Hartford Institute for Geriatric Nursing want to know more. 2012. Available at: http://consultgerirn.org/topics/critical_care/want_to_know_more. Accessed February 10, 2013.
5. Try this general assessment series. In: Hartford Institute of Geriatric Nursing. 2013. Available at: http://consultgerirn.org. Accessed January 8, 2013.
6. Hall GR, Maslow K. Working with families of hospitalized older adults with dementia. In: Try this: dementia series. 2007. Available at: http://consultgerirn.org. Accessed January 8, 2013.
7. Morandi A, McCurley J, Vasilevskis EE, et al. Tools to detect delirium superimposed on dementia: a systematic review. J Am Geriatr Soc 2012;60:2005–13.

8. Greenberg SA. The geriatric depression scale (GDS). In: Try this general assessment series. 2012. Available at: http://consultgerirn.org. Accessed January 8, 2013.
9. Shelkey M, Wallace M. Katz index of independence in activities of daily living (ADL). In: Try this general assessment series. 2012. Available at: http://consultgerirn.org. Accessed January 8, 2013.
10. Caceres BA, Fulmer T. Mistreatment detection. In: Boltz M, Capezuti E, Fulmer T, et al, editors. Evidence-based geriatric nursing protocols for best practice. 4th edition. New York: Springer; 2012. p. 544–52.
11. Caldwell HK, Gilden G, Meuller M. Elder abuse screening instruments in primary care: an integrative review, 2004 to 2011. Clin Geriatr 2013;21:20–5.
12. Johnson VB. Oral hygiene care for functionally dependent and cognitively impaired older adults. J Gerontol Nurs 2012;38:11–9. Available at: http://www.healio.com/nursing/journals/JGN. Accessed November 7, 2012.
13. Morritt Taub LF. The Kayser-Jones brief oral health status examination (BOHSE). In: Try this general assessment series. 2012. Available at: http://consultgerirn.org. Accessed January 29, 2013.
14. Servat JJ, Risco M, Nakasato YR, et al. Visual impairment in the elderly: impact on functional ability and quality of life. Clin Geriatr 2011;19:49–56.
15. Carolan Doerflinger DM. Mental status assessment of older adults: the Mini-Cog. In: Try this general assessment series. 2013. Available at: http://consultgerirn.org. Accessed January 29, 2013.
16. Vasilveskis EE, Morandi A, Boehm L, et al. Delirium and sedation recognition using validated instruments: reliability of bedside intensive care unit nursing assessments from 2007 to 2010. J Am Geriatr Soc 2011;59:S249–55.
17. Hoskins BL. Safe prescribing for the elderly. Nurse Pract 2011;36:47–52.
18. The American Geriatrics Society Expert Panel. American Geriatrics Society updated Beers criteria for potentially inappropriate medication use in older adults. J Am Geriatr Soc 2012;60:616–31.
19. Fulmer T. Elder mistreatment assessment. In: Try this general assessment series. 2012. Available at: http://consultgerirn.org. Accessed January 29, 2013.

Ethnogeriatrics in Critical Care

Sonya R. Hardin, PhD, RN, CCRN, NP-C

KEYWORDS

- Ethnogeriatrics • Culture • Diversity • Ethnicity

KEY POINTS

- Ethnogeriatrics is a geriatric subspecialty emphasizing the intersection of knowledge from the fields of aging, health, and ethnicity.
- One-third of the older population is expected to be from a minority category within the next 10 years.
- Cultural competence among critical care nurses will be required to meet the needs/preferences of a diverse older population.
- The nurse will need to be a life-long learner and to focus on the individual patient and not stereotypes, maintain mutual respect, and congruent care strategies with their cultural background and expectations.

INTRODUCTION

Critical care units care for a high percentage of older adults. The diversity of older adults over the age of 65 is estimated to increase in the next 10 years with one-third of US population to be from one of the 4 minority categories (Hispanic, Asian, African American, or American Indian/Alaska native). Projections include that the number of non-Hispanic Black elders will more than triple from about 2.8 million to nearly 10 million, representing an increase in the proportion of African American elders from 8.1% to 12.2%—a 50% increase. Asian and Pacific Islander elders will grow in number from about 820,000 in 2000 to 5.3 million by midcentury, representing 6.5% of all older adults. Hispanic elders will increase in numbers from just less than 2 million to more than13.4 million.[1] By 2028, the Administration on Aging[2] estimates that Hispanic elders will represent the largest racial/ethnic minority among older adults.

Each racial and ethnic group has subpopulations such as within the Hispanic or Latino populations; individuals may be Mexican Americans, Puerto Ricans, Cubans, as well as from the Dominican Republic, and South or Central America. Also, Asians may have origins from China, the Philippines, Japan, Vietnam, Laos, Cambodia, India, or other areas. Vast differences related to health beliefs and practices, health risks, family dynamics and care-giving, decision-making process and priorities, and responses to interventions exist in the subpopulations.[3–7]

No Disclosures or Conflicts of Interest.
East Carolina University, College of Nursing, 600 Moye Boulevard, Greenville, NC 27858, USA
E-mail address: srhardin7970@gmail.com

Crit Care Nurs Clin N Am 26 (2014) 21–30
http://dx.doi.org/10.1016/j.ccell.2013.10.009
0899-5885/14/$ – see front matter © 2014 Elsevier Inc. All rights reserved.
ccnursing.theclinics.com

ETHNOGERIATRICS

Ethnogeriatrics is the branch of gerontology that intersects the concepts of aging, health, and ethnicity.[8] However, before discussing ethnogeriatrics issues in critical care it is important to clarify terms. A variety of terms that are often used are culture, race, and ethnicity. Culture refers to a set of shared beliefs, values, and patterns of behavior of a group of people. The term ethnicity is preferred for this article because it is a broader concept that encompasses commonalities based on any of the following: national origin (eg, Russian), race (eg, Asian), religion (Catholic), or language (eg, German). It is important to recognize intraethnic diversity. Knowing there is much variation within groups as between them will mitigate the tendency to stereotype members.

Ethnicity is a critical variable in how the care experience is perceived and treated by the patient and family. Cultural factors mediate preferred patterns of interaction. For instance, the meaning of critical illness; whether a particular critical condition is stigmatized or accepted; ways in which symptoms are identified and interpreted; patterns of decision-making and preferences for end-of-life care; appropriate modes of expression of pain and discomfort; the use of rituals, traditional healers, healing practices, and whether dependency that accompanies an illness is disvalued or considered part of the normal cycle of life. Clearly, ethnicity merits care consideration in critical care to ensure optimal outcomes.

HEALTH RISKS AND HEALTH DISPARITIES

Most Black older persons have at least one chronic condition and many have multiple conditions. Among the most frequently occurring conditions among Black elderly in 2005 to 2007 were hypertension (84%), diagnosed arthritis (53%), all types of heart disease (27%), sinusitis (15%), diabetes (29%), and cancer (13%). The comparable figures for all older persons were hypertension (71%), diagnosed arthritis (49%), all types of heart disease (31%), sinusitis (14%), diabetes (18%), and cancer (22%).[9]

In 2008 the National Health Interview Survey reported that only 36% of Hispanic persons aged 65+ had received pneumococcal vaccination as compared with 64% of non-Hispanic Whites and 43.4% of non-Hispanic Blacks. Also, a significant difference in ethnic groups existed in that 9.2% of Hispanic persons aged 65+ needed help from other persons for personal care as compared wirh 5.7% for non-Hispanic Whites and 10.3% of non-Hispanic Blacks. Also of note, 10.7% of Hispanic persons aged 65+ were diagnosed with diabetes as compared with 6.9% for non-Hispanic Whites and 10.9% for non-Hispanic Blacks.[10]

There were differences by race and ethnicity in the prevalence of certain chronic health conditions. In 2009–2010, among people age 65 and over, non-Hispanic Blacks reported higher levels of hypertension and diabetes than non-Hispanic Whites (69% compared with 54% for hypertension, and 32% compared with 18% for diabetes). Hispanics also reported higher levels of diabetes (33%) than non-Hispanic Whites, but lower levels of arthritis (44% compared with 53%).[11]

Ethnic groups also differ in the impact of comorbid conditions on perceived appropriateness of intensive care admission. Considering intensive care units admission for persons with dementia, fewer than 50% of Anglos but more than 80% of Mexican Americans endorse such admissions.[12]

There are multiple complex systems of illness belief in each culture that affect the family and ethnic elders' illness behaviors, such as expression of pain and desired expected treatments.[13] All ethnic groups have indigenous health care systems that include methods of prevention, diagnosis, and treatment of health problems, as they are diagnosed by and for members of that group.

Beliefs regarding treatments and procedures in the intensive care unit may also vary by ethnic group. For example, beliefs regarding autopsy have been reported to vary dramatically between Anglos and Mexican Americans. In a recent study, Anglos reported that autopsies advanced science and improve patient care, whereas Mexican Americans contended that they offered no useful information unless they could help families understand a mysterious death. Furthermore, Mexican Americans reported that discussion of such decisions could be harmful, possibly hastening death. Finally, Anglos reported no harm coming to the deceased person from an autopsy, whereas Mexican Americans believed that the soul remains near the body and can feel the pain associated with the autopsy.[14]

The extent to which ethnic elders ascribe to these traditional belief systems and corresponding illness behaviors depends on multiple interacting factors, including the elder's generation of immigration, English-language proficiency, access to traditional and scientific practitioners, level of education, and gender. An understanding of the range of illness beliefs and cultural norms provides the basis for understanding patient and family responses to illness and treatment options.[15]

Having a strong knowledge base of the risk factors for disease by ethnic population among older adults as well as the health values and beliefs of the patients is critical for improving optimal outcomes.

CULTURAL COMPETENCE

Cultural competence has been highlighted in 2 Institute of Medicine reports, *Crossing the Quality Chasm*[16] and *Unequal Treatment*.[17] To eliminate racial disparities in health care, there is a need to reduce risk and improve patient adherence and health outcomes. A key aspect of cultural competence is providing respect for patient's values and to strive to provide services within their values, beliefs, norms, behaviors, and shared customs.

Although there exists commonalities among groups, one must always remember that cultural processes differ within the same group due to age, cohort, gender political climate, class religion ethnicity personality, sexual orientation, vocation, disability, language, immigration, and other factors. Respect for the patient and family should be ethnically appropriate while considering the amount of acculturation that has occurred with the patient living in America.

Nurses must have awareness of one's personal biases and how these biases can impact care. Cultural awareness involves the ability of becoming aware of one's own cultural values, beliefs, and perceptions. Misinterpretations occur when individuals do not ask what a behavior means to the patient.[18]

Becoming aware of our cultural dynamics is a difficult task because culture is not conscious to individuals. Since we are born, we have learned to see and do things at an unconscious level. Our experiences, our values, and our cultural background lead us to see and do things in a certain way. Sometimes we have to step outside of our cultural boundaries to realize the impact that our culture has on our behavior. It is very helpful to gather feedback from foreign colleagues on our behavior to get more clarity on our cultural traits.[19]

COMMUNICATION STRATEGIES

Using various communication strategies specifically designed to engage a culturally appropriate dialogue is necessary for care quality. **Box 1** lists several communication strategies from the literature that are useful with various ethnic groups.

Box 1
Communication strategies

- LEARN: Listen, Explain, Acknowledge, Recommend, Negotiate[20]
- PEARLS: Partnership, Empathy, Apology, Respect, Legitimization, Support[21]
- Six Steps of Culturally Informed Care[22]: (1) ethnic identity; (2) what is at stake?; (3) illness narrative; (4) stresses; (5) cultural influence on patient care and patient/provider relationship
- RISK Assessment: Resources, Individual identity, Skills to cope/adapt, Knowledge about ethnic groups[23]
- CRASH: Culture, Respect, Assess/affirm, Sensitive/self-awareness, Humility[24]
- QIAN: Self-questioning, Immersion, Active listening, Negotiation[25]
- 4 Cs of Culture: Call, Cause, Cope, Concerns[26]

During communication with ethnic elders, the nurse should consider the pace of conversation because some cultures used periods of silence and others may speak before the nurse finishes a sentence. Due to the various levels of acculturation, terms that are colloquial expressions should always be avoided. Observing the physical proximity of family to each other and to the nurse will provide information on the comfort level of individuals for the appropriate physical distance expected during conversations. Individuals from some cultures (eg, Northern European) tend to prefer to be about an arm's length away from another person, whereas those from some other cultures tend to prefer closer proximity (eg, some Hispanic/Latino cultures) or greater distance (eg, some Asian cultures). During conversation, some ethnic elders may consider eye contact disrespectful or impolite (eg, some Asian and Native American groups). Emotional expressiveness can vary among cultural groups, for example, older Japanese, Filipino, and Thai may laugh or smile to mask other emotions and Native Americans may express stoicism. During the process of communication, nurses should consider that body gestures could be misinterpreted as culturally inappropriate. Also, physical touch is highly variable across cultures and should not be used until nurses are debriefed about cultural appropriateness of touch. During a physical examination, a nurse should ask permission before touching or palpating to identify physical proximity and modesty issues.[27]

To communicate with ethnic elders with limited English proficiency, a nurse will need to obtain a trained interpreter.[28] Although the use of family members, especially the children of an elder, may seem convenient, this is discouraged due to the possible lack of appropriate language skills in one or both languages; culturally based modesty barriers to discussion of sensitive topics, especially across genders and age hierarchy, may lead to difficulty in discussing family problems.[29] Therefore, nurses can be the ethnic elders' advocate by obtaining on-site interpreter services and/or accessing telephone-based interpretation services.[30] Always explain to the patient and family that the use of a trained interpreter is facility policy to ensure clear communication.

Each approach can be useful for enhancing communication with ethnic elders. Nurses should chose an approach; often used is the LEARN model.[20] Berlin and Fowkes[20] created a cultural competency tool that provides guidelines in clinical practice for attending to issues in cross-cultural communication with patients. The tool is called LEARN. It consists of Listen, Explain, Acknowledge, Recommend, and Negotiate. Nurses should listen to the patient and family or other persons the elder relies on for health care advice. Listening with sympathy and understanding of the perception of the patient's problem is the first step. Questions to ask include, What do you think may be causing the problem?; How do you think the illness is affecting you? What do you think might be beneficial? After gathering information from the patient, the second step is to explain in the patient's language—at a level the patient can understand and in terms that are important to the patient—the possible diagnosis and steps that will be recommended for improving outcome of the condition. The nurse and providers should provide some preliminary explanation of what could be causing the problem. Next in the conversation, nurses should acknowledge the patient's understanding of their illness and bridge the gap between belief system of the patient and provider. Next, the nurse and provider should make a recommendation. Always after making a recommendation, the patient should be asked which strategy would be best. The patient should be involved in the decision-making of the treatment to ensure that culturally relevant approaches are incorporated. Critical to the success of a plan of care is to check for patient and family understanding and acceptance of the plan. Negotiating what the actual plan of care will be with either the patient or the decision-maker of the patient is more likely to ensure recovery.[20] The plan should fit within the cultural framework of the patient's perception. During the negotiation of the plan, it is especially important to acknowledge cultural differences and attempt to provide care to all patients in the same manner. For many ethnic older persons, the patient-clinician trust relationship is often influenced by cultural norms. Likewise, the clinical interaction is also impacted by the cultural background of health care providers.[31]

EXPLANATORY MODELS OF HEALTH

Nurses should validate the patient and family's explanations and expectations of the illness, which will enhance the providers' understanding of cultural beliefs. Questions that can help to uncover the explanatory model of an individual's illness were developed by Kleinman and colleagues.[26] Questions to ask include (1) What do you call the problem? (2) What do think has caused the problem? (3) Why do you think it started when it did? (4) What do you think the sickness does? How does it work? (5) How severe is the sickness? (6) What kind of treatment do you think the patient should receive? (7) What are the chief problems the sickness has caused? and (8) What do you fear most about the sickness?[32]

CULTURAL COMPETENCE TRAINING

Nurses should receive training in cultural competence and education on cultural groups treated in the region of their practice. Although it is unrealistic to expect a health professional to be proficient in working with every category and subgroup of minority older persons, it is possible to develop levels of awareness, skills, and sensitivity that can be applied to interactions with ethnic minority older persons and their families. Three important resources are (1) the Culture Med Ethnogeriatrics Overview (http://geriatrics.stanford.edu/culturemed/overview/introduction/); (2) the Curriculum in EthnoMed, which includes 5 background modules of a core curriculum in ethnogeriatrics and 13 ethnic-specific modules[18] (www.stanford.edu/group/ethnoger); (3) Doorway Thoughts: Cross-Cultural Health Care for Older Adults,[33] developed by the Ethnogeriatric Committee of the American Geriatrics Society, which includes 2 volumes of descriptions and relevant health concerns for 15 ethnic populations and a third volume featuring religious diversity; and (4) Ethnogeriatric and Cultural Competence for Nursing Practice (http://consultgerirn.org/topics/ethnogeriatrics_and_cultural_competence_for_nursing_practice/want_to_know_more).[34]

ETHNOGERIATRIC ASSESSMENT

Besides completing a standard assessment, nurses should also include an ethno-geriatric assessment. This assessment will specifically gather information for providing cultural-specific nursing care. Information on ethnicity, level of acculturation, religion/spirituality, preferred interaction patterns, facilitation of communication, and physical examination constraints should be collected to develop a plan of care.[35] A patient should be asked to self-identify his/her ethnicity. An older person may be classified by skin color, however, he may self-identify as a different ethnicity. Questioning the patient or family about the level of acculturation is important to provide a context for understanding the degree to which an ethnic older person has integrated the cultural beliefs, values, and practices of the mainstream society into her/his cultural beliefs and values.[25] Some indicators of acculturation that can be used quickly are (1) length of time the older patients or their ancestor has been in the United States and (2) language used at home, which gives some indication of fluency in spoken and written English.[26]

Information on affiliation with a specific religion or spiritual practice provides some information toward understanding their perspective of health. Also, a family's pattern of decision-making could be associated with religion, or culturally designated authority with the family. In some cultures, a trusted member of the ethnic community may be the preferred person to initiate a discussion about the care of the patient. This information will help the nurse and providers understand caregiving roles, and key individuals that are in a position to make health care decisions.[22]

Other clinical assessment domains to collect data on are the individuals' social history. Understanding the family and peer support my help to determine social isolation, risk for depression, and the availability of resources of the patient. A nurse caring for individuals in a critical care setting must be careful of terminology used with family members, because dementia and depression are considered mental illness in some cultures. Although dementia is considered a normal part of aging, in western culture it can be highly stigmatized.[21]

Box 2
Five key critical care nursing cultural competencies

1. Assess patient and family's position on the continuum of acculturation in relation to their preferences, perceptions, and definitions, and their explanatory models of physical and mental health and illness, their health literacy, and their health behaviors.

2. Demonstrate interviewing skills that promote culturally appropriate decision-making and mutual respect between health care providers and ethnic patients and their families.

3. Communicate effectively and elicit information from ethnic elders with appropriate use of interpreter services or oral and written strategies mindful of health literacy levels and abilities.

4. Identify available resources within older individuals, their families, and their ethnic communities for promoting and maintaining elders' physical, mental, and spiritual health, and support those resources in a respectful way.

5. Maintain up-to-date knowledge on health disparities in geriatric care and the effect of ethnicity and culture on physical and mental health care of older adults.

Adapted from Stanford Geriatric Education Center. Available at: http://sgec.stanford.edu/competencies.html.

ADVANCE DIRECTIVES AND END-OF-LIFE PREFERENCES

There is increasing attention on end-of-life care in health care systems. The health professional must strive to have an understanding of the ethnic older person's perspective about life and death and incorporate them into the care plan. The knowledge and understanding of advance directives vary among ethnic groups and subgroups. Talking

---

Box 3
The 2013 National CLAS standards

Principal standard

1. Provide effective, equitable, understandable, and respectful quality care and services that are responsive to diverse cultural health beliefs and practices, preferred languages, health literacy, and other communication needs.

Governance, leadership, and workforce

2. Advance and sustain organizational governance and leadership that promotes CLAS and health equity through policy, practices, and allocated resources.

3. Recruit, promote, and support a culturally and linguistically diverse governance, leadership, and workforce that are responsive to the population in the service area.

4. Educate and train governance, leadership, and workforce in culturally and linguistically appropriate policies and practices on an ongoing basis.

Communication and language assistance

5. Offer language assistance to individuals who have limited English proficiency and/or other communication needs, at no cost to them, to facilitate timely access to all health care and services.

6. Inform all individuals of the availability of language assistance services clearly and in their preferred language, verbally and in writing.

7. Ensure the competence of individuals providing language assistance, recognizing that the use of untrained individuals and/or minors as interpreters should be avoided.

8. Provide easy-to-understand print and multimedia materials and signage in the languages commonly used by the populations in the service area.

Engagement, continuous improvement, and accountability

9. Establish culturally and linguistically appropriate goals, policies, and management accountability and infuse them throughout the organization's planning and operations.

10. Conduct ongoing assessments of the organization's CLAS-related activities and integrate CLAS-related measures into assessment measurement and continuous quality improvement activities.

11. Collect and maintain accurate and reliable demographic data to monitor and evaluate the impact of CLAS on health equity and outcomes and to inform service delivery.

12. Conduct regular assessments of community health assets and needs and use the results to plan and implement services that respond to the cultural and linguistic diversity of populations in the service area.

13. Partner with the community to design, implement, and evaluate policies, practices, and services to ensure cultural and linguistic appropriateness.

14. Create conflict- and grievance-resolution processes that are culturally and linguistically appropriate to identify, prevent, and resolve conflicts or complaints.

15. Communicate the organization's progress in implementing and sustaining CLAS to all stakeholders, constituents, and the general public.[38]

about death is considered inappropriate in some cultures (eg, Chinese, Navajo); hence, the topic should be approached carefully and sensitively, and only in the context of an established trusting relationship. A possible introduction after several interactions might be, "In case something happens to you and you are not able to make decisions about your care, we will need to know your preferences." A direct approach about death may be too intrusive for some groups (eg, Filipino). A minister/priest known to the older person may bring up the subject, "When the time comes, what would you like your family and the health care providers do?" The family may be guided on how to bring up the subject. Other areas to explore include (1) preferred site for end-of-life care (ie, hospital or home), (2) cultural practices associated with care of the body and mourning behaviors during and after death, and (3) attitudes about organ donation and autopsy. The patient/family may think that cultural rituals and traditions practiced at the time of death may not be honored. Therefore, reassurance will be needed.[23,36,37] **Box 2** displays the 5 nursing competencies that should be used in the critical care unit to ensure culture-specific care is delivered to ethnic elders.

ORGANIZATIONAL INTEGRATION

The organization should develop policies to support and reward direct care providers to develop treatment plans guided by ethnogeriatric concepts and principles. The most important comprehensive step that health care organizations can take to provide competent ethnogeriatric care is to ensure that the 15 Culturally and Linguistically Appropriate Services (CLAS) standards (**Box 3**) developed by the Office of Minority Health are implemented. The 2013 National CLAS Standards emphasize the importance of CLAS being integrated throughout an organization. This integration requires a bottom-up and a top-down approach to advancing and sustaining CLAS. Organizational governance and leadership are key to ensuring the successful implementation and maintenance of CLAS.

SUMMARY

Over the past 15 years, an explosion of information on older minority health in professional literature and professional meetings has increased the availability of materials to develop the field further. Thus, the depth and reach of ethnogeriatrics will continue to evolve over time.[39]

Adapting to the changing demographics will go beyond the recognition of the racial/ethnic groupings reflected by the Census Bureau (White, Black or African American, American Indian or Alaska Native, Asian, and Native Hawaiian or Other Pacific Islander). The growth in the government's recognized ethnic groups does not begin to reflect the tremendous diversity that must be addressed in clinical care because of the within-group diversity found in each population.[40]

ACKNOWLEDGMENTS

The author wishes to acknowledge the faculty in the Stanford Geriatric Education Center (SGEC), in the Stanford University School of Medicine, for their support in the 2012–2013 intensive 12-month 160-hour Faculty Development Program in Ethnogeriatrics (FDPE). This article was developed as part of the program.

REFERENCES

1. US Census Bureau. 2010. Available at: http://www.census.gov/2010census/. Accessed September 16, 2013.

2. Administration on Aging. A statistical profile of Hispanic older Americans aged 65+. Washington, DC: Administration on Aging; 2007.
3. McBride M, Lewis I. African American and Asian American elders: an ethnogeriatric perspective. In: Fitzpatrick J, Villaruel A, Porter C, editors. Annual review for nursing research, vol. 2. New York: Springer Publishing Co., Inc; 2004. p. 161–214.
4. McBride MR, Morioka-Douglas N, Yeo G. Aging and health: Asian and Pacific Island American elders. SGEC Working Paper Series No. 3. 2nd edition. Stanford (CA): Stanford Geriatric Education Center; 1996.
5. McCabe M, Cuellar J. Aging and health: American Indian/Alaska Native elders. Ethnogeriatric Reviews: Working Paper Series No. 6. 2nd edition. Palo Alto (CA): Stanford Geriatric Education Center, Stanford University; 1994.
6. Richardson J. Aging and Health: Black American elders. SGEC Working Paper #4. 2nd edition. Stanford (CA): Stanford GEC; 1996.
7. Villa ML, Cuellar J, Gamel N, et al. Aging and health: Hispanic American elders. SGEC Working Paper #5. 2nd edition. Stanford (CA): Stanford GEC; 1993.
8. Klein S, editor. Ethnogeriatrics. In a national agenda for geriatric education: white papers. Washington, DC: Bureau of Health Professions, Health Resources and Services Administration; 1996.
9. Administration on Aging. A statistical profile of Black older Americans aged 65+. Washington, DC: Administration on Aging; 2010.
10. Pleis JR, Lucas JW, Ward BW. Summary health statistics for US adults: national health interview survey 2008. Vital Health Stat 10 2009;242:1–157.
11. Federal Interagency Forum on Aging Related Statistics. Health status. Available at: http://www.agingstats.gov/Main_Site/Data/2012_Documents/Health_Status.aspx. Accessed September 16, 2013.
12. Caralis PV, Davis B, Wright K, et al. The influence of ethnicity and race on attitudes toward advance directives, life-prolonging treatments, and euthanasia. J Clin Ethics 1993;4:155–65.
13. Haley WE, Han B, Henderson JN. Aging and ethnicity: issues for clinical practice. J Clin Psychol Med Settings 1998;5:393–409.
14. Perkins HS, Supik JD, Hazuda HP. Cultural differences among health professionals: a case illustration. J Clin Ethics 1998;9(2):108–17.
15. Kelly LS, Tripp-Reimer T, Choi E, et al. Ethnogeriatrics issues in critical care. Chapter 21. In: Fulmer TT, Foreman MD, Walker M, et al, editors. Critical care nursing of the elderly. 2nd edition. New York: Springer Publishing Company, Inc; 2001. p. 353–77.
16. Committee on Quality of Health Care in America, Institute of Medicine. Crossing the quality chasm: a new health system for the 21st century. Washington, DC: National Academy Press; 2001.
17. Smedley BD, Stith AY, Nelson AR, editors. Unequal treatment: confronting racial and ethnic disparities in health care. Washington, DC: National Academy Press; 2003.
18. Yeo G. Ethnogeriatric curriculum: core curriculum and ethnic specific modules. Collaborative on Ethnogeriatric Education; 2001. 2002 [on-line]. Available at: http://geriatrics.stanford.edu/ethnomed/. Accessed September 16, 2001.
19. Adler NJ. International dimensions of organizational behavior. 2nd edition. Boston: Kent Publishing; 1991.
20. Berlin EA, Fowkes WG. A Teaching framework for cross-cultural health care. Cross-Cultural Medicine. West J Med 1983;139:934–8.
21. Steele D, Harrison J. Challenging physician-patient interactions. Leawood (KS): American Academy of Family Physicians; 2002.

22. Kleinman A, Benson P. Anthropology in the clinic: the problem of cultural competency and how to fix it. PLoS Med 2006;3(10):e294.

23. Kagawa-Singer M, Kassim-Lakha S. A strategy to reduce cross-cultural miscommunication and increase the likelihood of improving health outcomes. Acad Med 2003;78(6):577–87.

24. Rust G, Kondwani K, Martinez R, Dansie R, Wong W, Fry-Johnson Y, et al. A crash-course in cultural competence. Ethn Dis 2006;16(Suppl 3):S3–29, 36.

25. Chang ES, Simon M, Dong XQ. Integrating cultural humility into health care professional education and training. Adv Health Sci Educ Theory Pract 2012; 17(2):269–78.

26. Galanti GA. Caring for patients from different cultures. Philadelphia: University of PA Press; 2008.

27. Yeo G, McBride M. Cultural diversity in gerontology and geriatrics education. In: Sterns HL, Bernard MA, Schaie W, editors. Annual review of gerontology and geriatrics, gerontological and geriatric education, vol. 28. New York: Springer; 2008. p. 93–109.

28. Diaz-Duque OF. Overcoming the language barrier: advice for an interpreter. Am J Nurs 1982;82:1380–2.

29. Jackson C. Medical interpretation. In: Loue S, editor. Handbook of immigrant health. New York: Plenum Press; 1998. p. 61–79.

30. Villarreul AM, Portillo CJ, Kane P. Communicating with limited English proficiency persons: implications for nursing practice. Nurs Outlook 1999;47:262–70.

31. Takeshita J, Ahmed I. Culture and geriatric psychiatry. In: Tseng WS, Streltzer J, editors. Cultural competence in clinical psychiatry. Washington, DC: American Psychiatric Publishing; 2004. p. 147–61.

32. Kleinman A, Eisenberg L, Good B. Culture, illness and care. Ann Intern Med 1978;88:251–8.

33. Adler R (Vol. 1 & 2) Adler R, Grudzen M (Vol. 3) eds. Doorway Thoughts: Cross-Cultural Health Care for Older Adults, Ethnogeriatric Committee of American Geriatric Society Sudbury, MA Jones & Bartlett 2004, 2006, 2008.

34. Mcbride M. Ethnogeriatric and cultural competence for nursing practice. 2012. Available at: http://consultgerirn.org/topics/ethnogeriatrics_and_cultural_competence_for_nursing_practice/want_to_know_more. Accessed September 16, 2013.

35. Mezey MD, Rauckhorst LH, Stokes SA. Health assessment of the older individual. New York: Springer Publishing Company; 1993. Evidence Level VI.

36. Yeo G. How will the U.S. health care system meet the challenge of the ethnogeriatric imperative? J Am Geriatr Soc 2009;57(7):1278–85.

37. Moon A, Lubben JE, Villa V. Awareness and utilization of community long-term care services by elderly Korean and Non-Hispanic white Americans. Gerontologist 1998;38(3):309–18.

38. US Department of Health and Human Services. National standards for culturally and linguistically appropriate services (CLAS) in health and health care. Office of Minority Health; 2013. Available at: https://www.thinkculturalhealth.hhs.gov/Content/clasvid.asp. Accessed October 31, 2013.

39. Werkmeiser-Rozas L, Klein WC. Cultural responsiveness in long-term-care case management: moving beyond competence. Care Manag J 2009;10(1):2–7.

40. Pardasani M. Senior centers: increasing minority participation through diversification. J Gerontol Soc Work 2004;43(2/3):41–56.

Nutrition and Hydration in Older Adults in Critical Care

Rose Ann DiMaria-Ghalili, PhD, RN, CNSC[a],*,
Michele Nicolo, MS, RD, CDE, CNSD, LDN[b]

KEYWORDS

- Critical illness • Nutrition assessment • Enteral nutrition • Parenteral nutrition
- Hydration • Older adults

KEY POINTS

- Older adults are vulnerable to alterations in nutrition and hydration during critical illness.
- The best way to address nutrition and hydration challenges during critical illness is through a unified approach with a multidisciplinary team consisting of physicians, nurses, dietitians, pharmacists, physical therapists, speech therapists, and respiratory therapists, as well as the patient and family caregiver.
- Nurses often provide one-to-one care for critically ill older adults and are in a unique position to promote nutrition and to monitor and evaluate the effectiveness of therapy.
- As the science and practice of gerontologic nursing expands to meet the needs of the increasing critically ill aging population, further research is needed to address nutrition and hydration in critically ill older adults.

INTRODUCTION

As the number of older adults continues to increase in the United States, so will those who require critical care during the course of hospitalization.[1] Experts predict that the largest proportion of beds in intensive care units (ICUs) will be occupied by older adults,[1] and the oldest old ($\geq$80 years) will account for in 1 in 4 admissions to the ICU.[2] Respiratory insufficiency/failure, postoperative management, ischemic heart disorder, sepsis, and heart failure are the most common reasons for ICU admissions[3] and are likely to continue as more older adults are admitted to the ICU. In order to improve outcomes of critically ill older adults, ICU nurses must address the unique needs of the older adult during critical illness.

Disclose any Relationship: R.A. DiMaria-Ghalili received honorarium from Nestle Health Institute in the past year to deliver an educational presentation.
[a] Doctoral Nursing Department, College of Nursing and Health Professions, Drexel University, 245 North 15th Street, Mail Stop 1030, Philadelphia, PA 19102, USA; [b] Clinical Nutrition Support Services, Hospital of the University of Pennsylvania, 1912 Penn Tower, 1 Convention Avenue, Philadelphia, PA 19104, USA
* Corresponding author.
E-mail address: rad83@drexel.edu

Crit Care Nurs Clin N Am 26 (2014) 31–45
http://dx.doi.org/10.1016/j.ccell.2013.10.006
0899-5885/14/$ – see front matter © 2014 Elsevier Inc. All rights reserved.

Nutrition and fluid balance are vital components of critical care nursing. However, meeting the nutrition and hydration needs of the critically ill older adult is often complex because of preexisting risk factors (malnutrition, unintentional weight loss, frailty, and dehydration); as well as ICU-related challenges (catabolism, eating and feeding, end-of-life care). This article highlights the challenges of managing nutrition and hydration in the critically ill older adult, reviews assessment principles, and offers strategies for optimizing nutrition and hydration.

PREEXISTING NUTRITION AND HYDRATION CHALLENGES
Malnutrition

Before even entering the ICU, older adults are at risk for malnutrition (undernutrition), because of dietary, economic, psychosocial, and physiologic factors.[4] Malnutrition is associated with increased costs, as well as adverse health outcomes, which include poor wound healing, infections, postoperative complications, increased length of stay, prolonged mechanical ventilation, and mortality.[4–8] Although 12% to 72% of hospitalized older adults have malnutrition, or are at risk for malnutrition,[6] little is known about the prevalence of malnutrition in older adults on admission to the ICU. Recently, Sheean and colleagues[9] reported the prevalence of malnutrition in older adults admitted to a medical or surgical ICU at 23% to 34% using the Mini-Nutrition Assessment (MNA), Subjective Global Assessment, and Nutrition Risk Score 2002. Older adults who are already at nutritional risk can have a rapid decline in nutritional status during an ICU stay if appropriate nutritional interventions are not implemented in a timely fashion.

UNINTENTIONAL WEIGHT LOSS

Unintentional weight loss is not a normal part of aging,[10] and can occur in isolation[11] or as a component of geriatric syndromes such as malnutrition (undernutrition),[12] frailty,[13] as well as sarcopenia,[14] cachexia,[14] and inflammatory conditions.[14] Unintentional weight loss is associated with hospital readmissions[15,16] and falls[17,18] and increases the risk for death.[19–21] The danger of weight loss in older adults is the loss of lean mass or muscle, which results in a decline in functional status.[10,22–24] A weight loss of 5% of usual body weight during 6 to 12 months is the most widely accepted definition for clinically important weight loss in noninstitutionalized older adults.[25] Interventions primarily focus on treating risk factors for unintentional weight loss, as well as optimizing nutritional intake.[26,27] Appetite stimulants may be used in older adults with unintentional weight loss in long-term care settings,[26] but there is little guidance regarding their use during the critical care phase of the illness trajectory.

Frailty

The prevalence of preexisting frailty in critically ill older adults is unknown; however, experts suggest that it will likely increase as more older adults are admitted to the ICU.[28] Frailty is defined as "a biological syndrome of decreased reserve and resistance to stressors, resulting from cumulative declines across multiple physiological systems, and causing vulnerability to adverse outcomes."[13(ppM146)] Frailty exists when at least 3 of the following symptoms are present: weakness, slow walking speed, low physical activity, unintentional weight loss, and exhaustion.[29] Older adults who present to the ICU with frailty have poor physiologic reserve and may not withstand the increased physiologic demands from the underlying critical illness. Frail older adults can have a rapid decline in their functional status, leading to disability and prolonged recovery time after critical illness. Recently, McDermid and colleagues[28] suggested that the issue with frailty in critically ill older adults is not only because of the chronic nature of the preexisting condition but is also the result of the acute critical care state, which can overwhelm reserves, leading to muscle wasting, weakness, and poor functional status, even after discharge from the ICU. Interventions to combat frailty in the ICU include optimizing nutrition support, sedation interruption, early mobilization, and preventing physical disability with physical therapy.[28] Further research is needed to evaluate the impact of frailty interventions[30] on ICU outcomes.

DEHYDRATION

Older adults are at risk for dehydration because of mobility and functional disabilities, incontinence, chronic illness, medications, air-fluidized beds, vomiting, diarrhea, fever and acute infections, burns, blood volume loss, tube feeding, nasogastric tube drainage, fistula drainage, and high-output ostomies.[31–33] Dehydration is one of the Agency for Healthcare Research and Quality's Prevention Quality Indicators (PQIs).[34] As a PQI, dehydration at hospital admission is a measure of ambulatory care sensitive conditions.[34] Dehydration occurs more frequently in older adults. In 2009, the rate of dehydration per 100,000 hospital admissions was 274.4 in the 65-year to 74-year age group and 709.35 in the ≥75-year age group.[35] Dehydration is associated with hospital admissions, functional decline, delirium, pressure ulcers, infection, falls, constipation, medication toxicity, increased length of stay and health care costs, and mortality.[33,36,37] Clearly, many older adults are likely to be dehydrated on admission to the ICU. Interventions focus on correcting the fluid imbalance and any associated hemodynamic instability.

ICU Issues Related to Nutrition and Hydration

Catabolic state

Acute and chronic inflammation is associated with decreased energy intake, decrease in weight, and decline in physical function.[38,39] Critically ill patients are catabolic because of the hypermetabolism associated with the acute-phase inflammatory response triggered from the underlying disease state.[40–42] This catabolic state increases not only energy needs but also protein needs because of nitrogen losses and breakdown of lean body mass.[41,43] Muscle breakdown occurs in order to provide an energy source for acute-phase proteins.[20,21] Energy and protein requirements are often increased with injury severity (ie, postoperative period and sepsis).[44] The inflammation of aging and chronic disease states can also play a role in the catabolic response during critical illness.[41,45,46] Also, critically ill older adults are confined to prolonged bed rest, which causes the breakdown of lean body mass, resulting in muscle wasting.[47] Although further research is needed to elucidate the impact of aging (which can span 40 years) on hypermetabolism and the acute-phase inflammatory response during critical illness, nutritional therapies need to be instituted in a timely fashion to thwart further nutritional and functional decline.

EATING AND FEEDING ISSUES

During hospital admission, achieving optimal oral nutrition intake may be an issue. Barriers to adequate oral intake include missing orders for diets, frequent nil-by-mouth orders for testing or procedures, restrictive diets, intolerance of food consistency, inability to chew food, dislike of hospital food, nausea and vomiting, lack of appetite, and the need for assistance with tray setup and feeding.[47,48] Eating less than 75% of daily calorie requirements can contribute to weight loss.[7,8] A large international study on nutrition screening reported an increase in 30-day mortality in those patients who consumed the least amount of calories on the day of data collection.[49] These barriers can also contribute to inadequate oral intake in the ICU and can worsen the degree of malnutrition.[7] Extubated patients are at particular risk for inadequate oral intake.[8] Tube feedings are usually discontinued after extubation if the gastrointestinal tract is functional. Peterson and colleagues[8] reported that energy and protein intake during the first 7 days after extubation never exceeded 55% of daily requirements. Although the researchers discussed general weakness and restrictive diets as potential reasons for decreased oral intake after extubation, they did not discuss alterations in swallowing or throat pain after extubation as contributing factors for decreased oral intake. The American Association of Critical Care Nurses' *Practice Alert for Prevention of Aspiration* recommends that patients should be assessed for swallowing problems, usually by a speech pathologist, before introduction of oral feedings in the postextubation period.[50] Diet modifications should then be implemented until swallowing problems are resolved. Although throat pain after prolonged intubation usually subsides within an hour after extubation,[51] those with persistent throat pain may also need diet modifications (ie, soft diet) until the pain resolves.

End-of-Life Issues

Before admitting an older adult to the ICU, their preferences regarding life-sustaining treatment should be determined.[52] However, there are times when the goal of ICU care becomes palliative, as opposed to curative or restorative. In these situations, the issue of artificial nutrition and hydration at end of life must be addressed with the older adult or surrogate. Providers should use their best clinical judgment when deciding to initiate tube feeding. The American Society for Parenteral and Enteral Nutrition's (ASPEN) *Ethics Position Paper* states that "health care professionals should not be ethically obligated to offer artificial nutrition and hydration if in their clinical judgment there is not adequate evidence for the therapy, or the burden or risk of the intervention far outweighs its benefit."[53(pp12)] Before tube feeding is started, the patient's wishes and advanced directives should be reviewed.[54] A discussion should take place with the patient or surrogate regarding the treatment goals for tube feeding (curative, rehabilitative, or palliative) as well as the anticipated outcome of providing or withholding tube feeding.[54]

Screening, Assessment, and Diagnoses

Screening
Nutrition screening is defined as a process to identify an individual who may be malnourished or at risk for malnutrition to determine if a detailed nutrition assessment is indicated.[55] In the hospital setting, the Joint Commission[56] mandates that every patient admitted to the hospital should have a nutrition screen performed within 24 hours of admission. In most settings, the initial nutrition screen is performed by nurses.[57] There are no standards that mandate a nutrition screen on admission to the ICU outside the first 24 hours of hospital admission. However, nutrition screening and rescreening can be performed by any health care professional using valid and reliable tools for older adults[58] and should be incorporated into the initial ICU assessment. More than 21 different nutrition screening and assessment tools have been developed for older adults[59]; however, most lack adequate validity and reliability. The Hartford Institute for Geriatric Nursing's *Best Practices in Nursing Care to Older Adults Try This* recommends the MNA (http://www.mna-elderly.com/) for use in older adults.[60] The MNA (full or short form) is the only screening (MNA–short form) and assessment tool (MNA–full form) that has been validated and used in more than 200 studies,[61] but there are limited studies using this tool in critically ill older adults.[9] Further

identification of the most appropriate data elements to incorporate into ICU nutrition screening tools, as well as validation of current nutrition screening tools for use in older patients in the ICU, should be performed.

Assessment

The goal of a nutrition assessment is to diagnose nutrition problems[55] and identify areas for further nutrition intervention.[62] Components include past and current medical/surgical history, medication history, adequacy of usual oral intake, weight history, laboratory data, physical examination, functional status, and psychosocial status.[63] During the assessment, it is important to identify any barriers to meeting calorie and protein needs.[64] Review current and past medical and surgical history to identify conditions that either increase nutritional requirements or compromise the intake, absorption, or metabolism of nutrients. Note any current conditions or injuries associated with an acute inflammatory response (eg, major infection/sepsis, adult respiratory distress syndrome, systemic inflammatory response syndrome, severe burns, major abdominal surgery, multiple trauma or closed head injury).[41] A history of the following conditions may predispose the older adult to nutritional alterations: previous gastrointestinal surgery, hemorrhage, or obstruction; enterocutaneous fistula; acute or chronic pancreatitis, inflammatory bowel disease, malignancy, organ failure/transplant, or AIDS.[41] Older adults are more likely to present with multiple comorbid chronic conditions that are managed by many medications.[64] Polypharmacy can interfere with food intake and can often cause issues with nausea, anorexia, dry mouth, change in taste of food, fullness, and nutrient absorption.[4,64]

The adequacy of oral intake should also be determined. However, if the patient is not eating, then normal dietary intake patterns should be determined by interviewing the patient or family or through review of the medical record. If the patient is eating, then dietary intake can be assessed with a modified diet history, 24-hour food recall,[65] or a calorie count.[4] However, recall methods may be inaccurate in those older adults with cognitive impairment.

Weight is a critical vital sign in older adults. In the ICU, weight should be measured on a daily basis using bed scales. Body mass index (BMI, calculated as weight in kilograms divided by the square of height in meters) is an indicator of body fatness, but it does not provide an accurate representation in sarcopenia and those with edema. The 1998 National Heart, Lung, and Blood Institute recommendation for a healthy BMI is 18.5 to 24.9 kg/m^2 for all adults.[66] There are several different recommendations for normal BMI for older adults. The 2002 Nutrition Screening Initiative recommends a healthy BMI of 22 to 27 for older adults.[67] The Centers for Medicare and Medicaid Services defines a normal BMI in older adults as 23 or higher and less than 30.[68] The percentage of weight change from baseline should be calculated (baseline or usual weight − current weight/100).[69] If an individual cannot recall if they lost weight, ask about changes in clothing size, examination of the belt, or ask significant others.[25] Because older adults may lose height as part of normal aging,[4] it is important to measure height. In the ICU, alternatives to standing height include demispan measurement,[4,41] or knee-height with a caliper.[4,65]

Albumin and prealbumin are visceral proteins, which were traditionally used to diagnose malnutrition. However, because negative acute-phase proteins, albumin, and prealbumin levels decrease during inflammation,[41,43,70] in order to determine if the depleted measures of albumin and prealbumin reflect malnutrition, it is recommended to monitor inflammatory markers such as C-reactive protein[65] or interleukin 6.[41] If these inflammatory markers are increased and albumin and prealbumin levels are low, then the changes in albumin and prealbumin are caused by an underlying inflammation.[65]

Physical assessment should focus on signs of muscle loss, fat loss, and presence of micronutrient deficiencies.[63] Loss of muscle and fat mass may be apparent, with bilateral temporal wasting, clavicular wasting, and loss of muscle tone in the extremities. Loss of muscle may be less apparent in obesity; however, techniques (skin-folds and circumferences) used to measure loss of muscle and fat may not be feasible in the critically ill population.[64] Poor dentition or ill-fitting dentures can prevent food from adequately being chewed, making mealtime more of an issue. Sensory loss of taste and smell can cause food to be less appealing. Older adults having pain or difficulty swallowing may avoid foods associated with these issues and in turn eliminate some macronutrients and micronutrients from their diet. Any difficulty with swallowing should be identified and further evaluated by a speech pathologist.[44,71]

Malnutrition can negatively affect muscle strength and muscle mass, leading to functional decline, frailty, and physical disability. Hand grip strength, an indicator of upper body muscle function, is used as an outcome variable in nutrition intervention studies as well as a marker of nutritional status.[72] Hand grip strength measurements are noninvasive, portable, and can easily be measured at the bedside[73] in those critically ill older adults who are responsive and able.[41] Functional limitations related to shopping, cooking, and eating should also be assessed.[4] An understanding of the home environment and social issues can shed light on factors that impede access to food as well as limited income to purchase food foods.[64] Depression and dementia can also cause decreased dietary intake, resulting in weight loss and eventual malnutrition.[4]

Fluid status

Both dehydration and overhydration (edema) should be assessed. Signs and symptoms of dehydration include poor skin turgor, sunken eyes, dry tongue with longitudinal furrows, dry skin and mucus membranes, muscle weakness and cramps, severe confusion, impaired speech, poor skin turgor, orthostatic blood pressure changes, light-headedness, and orthostasis and thirst.[31–33,74,75] In the ICU, intake and output should be monitored to determine fluid balance over time, and the impact of diuretics on fluid balance should also be considered.[76] Central venous pressure (CVP) readings may provide an indicator of hydration, but pulmonary stenosis and right ventricular failure can affect CVP measurements.[76] The presence of general or localized edema should also be assessed, paying particular attention to fluid accumulation in extremities, vulva/scrotum, or ascites[69] Edema can mask weight loss in malnourished individuals.[69]

Diagnosis

The purpose of nutrition screening and assessment is to identify findings to support a malnutrition (undernutrition) diagnosis. Over the years, researchers and clinicians have used a variety of clinical characteristics to define malnutrition. Inflammation has long been recognized as having a negative impact on nutrition status, because of breakdown of skeletal muscle,[77] and is now the cornerstone of the new adult malnutrition classification. Adult malnutrition is now identified as starvation-related malnutrition (caused by social or environmental circumstances, such as anorexia nervosa, alcoholism, lack of access to food); chronic disease-related malnutrition (inflammation of a mild to moderate degree, such as organ failure, pancreatic cancer, rheumatoid arthritis, and sarcopenic obesity); and acute disease-related malnutrition (acute inflammation with a marked inflammatory response, such as a major infection, burns, trauma, closed head injury).[23] The Academy of Nutrition and Dietetics and ASPEN issued a joint consensus document on specific criteria to diagnose these 3 types of malnutrition.[69] Patients must present with 2 of the following criteria in order to be diagnosed with malnutrition: inadequate/reduced energy intake, unintentional weight loss, loss of muscle mass, loss of fat mass, presence of edema or fluid accumulation, and a decrease in functional status as defined by reduced grip strength. These criteria reinforce the need for a comprehensive nutrition assessment, including a thorough nutrition history and an in-depth physical assessment, to identify signs of malnutrition.

Dehydration is considered a complex condition of reduced total body water from either a water deficit (eg, hypernatremia or hyponatremia with hyperglycemia) or both a salt and water deficit.[78] Biomarkers for dehydration include hematologic indices (serum sodium, blood urea nitrogen/creatinine ratio, and serum osmolality), and urinary indices (color-standardized chart and specific gravity).[33] However, serum osmolality is considered the gold standard to diagnosing dehydration.[33]

Interventions: Nutrient and Fluid Requirements

Nutrition needs for older adults differ only slightly from young adults. Older adults may not require as many calories because of reduced muscle mass and lower metabolic rate, but this can change in the setting of severe catabolism. However, overfeeding (providing an excess number of calories compared with energy expenditure) is detrimental, resulting in hyperglycemia, fatty liver, and excess carbon dioxide production.[52] Macronutrient needs, with the exception of protein, are similar to those of younger patients. Caloric requirements can be calculated using equations or through indirect calorimetry. The percentage of calories from carbohydrate and fat need to be adjusted accordingly based on patient needs. Older adults generally require more protein, but as liver and renal function decline with aging, higher protein intake should be closely monitored. Protein requirements range from 1 to 1.3 g/kg depending on the patient's needs. In addition to protein, older patients may also have increased micronutrient needs because of decreased gastrointestinal absorption.[79]

Fluid requirements can be estimated with 2 common methods: 1 mL of fluid for every kilocalorie consumed or 30 mL of fluid for every kilogram of body weight.[31,32] In an acute care setting, it is important to monitor fluid intake and output to determine hydration status and changes in electrolytes.[44] Some clinical situations may require higher hydration needs. Fluid losses related to vomiting, diarrhea, fistula drainage, and increased urine output may require more fluid intake to replace loss.[80] Patients who are febrile require additional hydration for insensible losses. On the other hand, fluid restriction may be indicated for patients with heart failure, renal issues, and those on diuretics.[44]

Initiating nutrition support

Before initiating any nutrition intervention, the critically ill older adult must be adequately resuscitated,[42] because shock states limit the use of nutrients.[40] Criteria to consider before starting nutrition interventions include completion of fluid resuscitation, mean arterial pressure, oxygen consumption, stable pressor agents, CVP, and serum lactate and base excess levels.[42] Feeding patients who require vasopressor medications is often debated. Feeding the gastrointestinal tract increases the need for oxygen.[81] Reduced blood flow to the gastrointestinal tract as a result of hypotension may result in an ischemic injury.[80] Once a patient has undergone fluid resuscitation and vasoactive medications are stable, enteral nutrition may be safely tolerated.[46]

Critically ill patients who have a functioning gastrointestinal tract and are able to take nutrients by mouth should be on an oral diet. To promote oral intake, dietary restrictions should be lifted when possible.[7] High-calorie snacks and supplements should be offered to increase the amount of calorie and protein consumed.[7]

Aggressive nutrition therapy should be considered if patients are consistently tolerating less than 50% to 75% of meals.[82] Patients with a history of anorexia, cognitive deficits, impaired gastrointestinal function, difficulty swallowing, and mechanical ventilation can preclude oral intake.[6] Nutrition support should be considered for patients who cannot meet their estimated nutrient needs orally.

Practice Guidelines

ASPEN publishes evidence-based practice standards on all components of enteral and parenteral therapies (http://www.nutritioncare.org). Although ASPEN does not have specific guidelines for older adults, the European Society for Parenteral and Enteral Nutrition (ESPEN) does (http://www.espen.org/education/espen-guidelines). Future guidelines need to address the unique characteristics of the older adult.

Enteral Nutrition

Enteral nutrition should be started in ICU patients when oral intake is not expected to be advanced within 24 to 48 hours.[44,83–85] Enteral nutrition is the preferred route for nutrition to maintain gut integrity and is associated with decreased length of stay and reduced infections and complications.[84,86,87] According to ASPEN's *Enteral Practice Recommendations,* patients' age, existing comorbidities, current nutrition risks, nutrient requirements, and available enteral access need to be assessed before starting enteral nutrition.[85] Providing 60% to 70% of estimated needs seems to have beneficial outcomes. Enteral nutrition may be contraindicated in situations such as severe gastrointestinal bleeding or ischemia, short bowel syndrome, significant malabsorption, high-output fistula, bowel obstruction or ileus, and inability to gain gastrointestinal access.[82,88] Factors to consider when selecting the type of formula include fluid status, presence or absence of organ failure, source of macronutrients, micronutrients, and malabsorption.[42] A 1-calorie-per-mL and high-protein formula is appropriate for most ICU patients. However, a more calorically dense formula (1.5–2.0 calories per mL) may be more appropriate in those patients who are fluid restricted or cannot tolerate a large volume of formula. A formula with a higher proportion of branched-chain amino acids may be appropriate for those patients in liver failure with refractory encephalopathy.[42] Although renal failure formulas contain more essential amino acids and lower levels of minerals and electrolytes, most patients with renal failure who are on hemodialysis or renal replacement therapy can tolerate a standard formula.[42] Patients in pulmonary failure may benefit from a formula that has less carbohydrate content and more fat. Fiber formulas should not be used in patients with bowel ischemia, but can be appropriate in those patients with malassimilation or diarrhea.[42] Some experts recommend the use of arginine-containing formulas for critically ill patients undergoing major surgery, trauma, or burns and those with head/neck cancer.[42] Peptide-based formulas or those with medium-chain triglycerides (MCTs) may be appropriate for patients with malabsorption, and antiinflammatory formulas for those with acute respiratory distress syndrome.[42]

Patients on enteral nutrition are at increased risk for dehydration if additional fluids are not administered. Enteral formulas contain between 70% and 90% free water, and more concentrated formulas have less free water.[89] Nurses can administer additional free water, especially during medication administration, through the feeding tube to achieve the daily fluid goal.

Parenteral Nutrition

Parenteral nutrition should be considered in those patients who cannot meet their nutrition needs via the enteral route. Risks associated with parenteral nutrition include electrolyte imbalances, hyperglycemia, hypertriglyceridemia, and infection.[90,91] Insulin resistance associated with critical illness and use of medications such as steroids and catecholamine contribute to an altered glycemic response.

The dextrose load in parenteral nutrition can exacerbate blood glucose levels and may increase the requirement for intravenous insulin infusion. Inability to obtain glycemic control can make it less likely that patients will be able to receive adequate calories in addition to causing other complications, such as risk for infection and delayed wound healing.[90,91]

Hydration status for patients receiving parenteral nutrition needs to be closely monitored. Depending on compounding practices, fluid requirements could be met via parenteral nutrition or the formula may be maximally concentrated, meaning that additional fluid has not been added to the bag. In this case, additional fluid may be required through intravenous infusions. For patients with glycemic control issues, saline solutions or lactated Ringer solution may be a better option than dextrose solutions; conversely, patients with hypernatremia or electrolyte abnormalities may require additional fluids in the form of dextrose solution. Monitoring clinical signs and symptoms, including urine output, blood pressure, and presence of edema, may provide insight into fluid needs.

Monitoring and Evaluation

Patient monitoring is necessary in order to adjust the nutrition regimen according to changes in clinical status.[70] This monitoring may include fluid status, electrolyte monitoring, and gastrointestinal tolerance. Daily weights and strict intake and output are important components of nursing care and provide essential information regarding the evaluation of nutrition care. Monitoring trends in weight provides insight into weight loss or weight gain because of fluid. Fluid accumulation, which is more common in the ICU patient, could mask weight and muscle loss. Patients who are volume overloaded may require a concentrated enteral or parenteral formula in order to provide optimal calorie and protein intake, with less volume.[80]

Older adults often present with multiple comorbidities, which may be exacerbated by an acute illness.[44] Regardless of the route of nutrition support, underlying chronic illnesses can add complexity to selecting the most appropriate formula. Electrolytes, blood glucose, and gastrointestinal symptom monitoring are vital to determining if low electrolyte formula, reduced dextrose/carbohydrate load, or an elemental or semielemental formula is indicated.[80] Refeeding syndrome may occur in malnourished patients with prolonged inadequate intake. Once nutrition support is started, patients should be carefully monitored for electrolyte imbalances (especially hypophosphatemia), arrhythmias, and changes in respiratory status.[80]

Nutrition support protocols and algorithms result in a better optimization of calorie and protein intake by influencing early feeding, with fewer interruptions.[83] Protocols (eg, clogged feeding tubes, gastric residual, and glycemic control) promote an interdisciplinary approach to patient care and enable nurses to make clinical decisions as complications arise.[92,93] Tube feeding protocols developed from evidence-based practice guidelines promote early initiation of nutrition support and increase delivery of calorie and protein.[83,92,93] Nurses play an important role in evaluating the patient's tolerance to enteral feedings. Methods to determine tolerance to gastric feeding include checking gastric residual volume (GRV) every 4 hours in gastrically fed patients.[85] If the GRV is 250 mL or higher after second GRV, a promotility agent should be considered.[85] If GRV is greater than 500 mL, tube feeds should be held and patient tolerance assessed (physical assessment, gastrointestinal assessment, glycemic control).[85] In addition, consider minimizing sedation and introduce a promotility agent.[85] When possible, feeding tubes should be positioned below the ligament of Treitz when GRVs are consistently measured greater than 500 mL.[85] The aspirated GRV should be returned to the stomach and not discarded.[94] Metheny and colleagues[95] recently surveyed the practices of critical care nurses and found that only 12% of respondents held tube feedings for a GRV of 500 mL or greater. Withholding enteral feeding for lower GRV volumes affects the overall nutrient delivery and nutritional status. Tube feeding patients should be monitored closely for aspiration risk, and nurses need to be vigilant in maintaining the head of the bed at 30° to 45° in patients receiving tube feeding.[85,96] Patients on enteral nutrition may have increased stool output or diarrhea. Sorbitol in liquid medications can often cause diarrhea, because of the higher osmotic load. Increased stool output is often attributed to starting enteral nutrition. Antibiotic therapy or *Clostridium difficile* infections are other reasons.[96] Calorically dense formulas or concentrated formulas have a higher osmotic load and can also cause diarrhea in tube-fed patients.[96] Interventions for diarrhea include removing sorbitol from liquid medications, obtaining stool cultures to rule out infectious diarrhea, initiating opiates after infectious cause has been ruled out, considering switching to formula with fiber or small peptides/MCTs, and adding additional fiber to formula.[42] Enteral nutrition is the preferred mode of nutrition support when the gastrointestinal tract is functional. However, patients frequently have their enteral nutrition interrupted because of availability of feeding pumps on the unit, perceived patient intolerance (abdominal distention, high gastric residuals, and vomiting), and the inability to maintain head of bed elevation at 30° to 45°. Frequent interruptions in feeding result in reduced calorie and protein intake.[83,92,97–99] Nurses need to be vigilant in minimizing the amount of time that tube feeding is interrupted.

In addition to monitoring tolerance to enteral and parenteral nutrition therapies, it is important to evaluate the impact of nutrition support. Even with adequate nutrition, it is difficult to reverse malnutrition during an acute inflammatory response. Goals of nutrition care for critically ill older adults should focus not only on decreasing the systemic inflammatory response and promoting an earlier return to physiologic baseline,[42] but also minimizing weight loss, preventing further nutritional decline, and restoration to baseline functional status.

SUMMARY

Older adults are vulnerable to alterations in nutrition and hydration during critical illness. The best way to address nutrition and hydration challenges during critical illness is through a unified approach with a multidisciplinary team consisting of physicians, nurses, dietitians, pharmacists, physical therapists, speech therapists, and respiratory therapists, as well as the patient and family caregiver. Nurses often provide one-to-one care for critically ill older adults and are in a unique position to promote nutrition and to monitor and evaluate the effectiveness of therapy. As the science and practice of gerontologic nursing expands to meet the needs of the increasing critically ill aging population, further research is needed to address nutrition and hydration in critically ill older adults.

REFERENCES

1. US Department of Health and Human Services. Health Resource Services Administration. Report to Congress. The critical care workforce: a study of the supply and demand for critical care physicians. Available at: http://bhpr.hrsa.gov/healthworkforce/reports/studycriticalcarephys.pdf. Accessed March 3, 2013.

2. Bagshaw SM, Webb SA, Delaney A, et al. Very old patients admitted to intensive care in Australia and New Zealand: a multi-centre cohort analysis. Crit Care 2009;13:R45.
3. Society of Critical Care Medicine. Critical care statistics in the United States. Available at: http://www.sccm.org/Communications/Pages/CriticalCareStats.aspx. Accessed November 3, 2013.
4. DiMaria-Ghalili RA, Amella E. Nutrition in older adults. Am J Nurs 2005;105(3):40.
5. Fry DE, Pine M, Jones BL, et al. Patient characteristics and the occurrence of never events. Arch Surg 2010;145:148.
6. Heersink JT, Brown CJ, Dimaria-Ghalili RA, et al. Undernutrition in hospitalized older adults: patterns and correlates, outcomes, and opportunities for intervention with a focus on processes of care. J Nutr Elder 2010;29:4.
7. Peterson SJ, Sheean PM, Braunschweig CL. Orally fed patients are at high risk of calorie and protein deficit in the ICU. Curr Opin Clin Nutr Metab Care 2011;14:182.
8. Peterson SJ, Tsai AA, Scala CM, et al. Adequacy of oral intake in critically ill patients 1 week after extubation. J Am Diet Assoc 2010;110:427.
9. Sheean PM, Peterson SJ, Chen Y, et al. Utilizing multiple methods to classify malnutrition among elderly patients admitted to the medical and surgical intensive care units (ICU). Clin Nutr 2013;32(5):752–7.
10. Miller SL, Wolfe RR. The danger of weight loss in the elderly. J Nutr Health Aging 2008;12:487.
11. Wallace JI, Schwartz RS. Epidemiology of weight loss in humans with special reference to wasting in the elderly. Int J Cardiol 2002;85:15.
12. Institute of Medicine. Retooling for an aging America. Washington DC: National Academies Press; 2010.
13. Fried LP, Tangen CM, Walston J, et al. Frailty in older adults: evidence for a phenotype. J Gerontol A Biol Sci Med Sci 2001;56:M146.
14. Thomas DR. Unintended weight loss in older persons. Aging Health 2008;4:191.
15. DiMaria-Ghalili RA. Changes in body mass index and late postoperative outcomes in elderly coronary bypass grafting patients: a follow-up study. Biol Res Nurs 2004;6:24.
16. Friedmann JM, Jensen GL, Smiciklas-Wright H, et al. Predicting early nonelective hospital readmission in nutritionally compromised older adults. Am J Clin Nutr 1997;65:1714.
17. Bales CW, Ritchie CS. Sarcopenia, weight loss, and nutritional frailty in the elderly. Annu Rev Nutr 2002;22:309.
18. Zoltick ES, Sahni S, McLean RR, et al. Dietary protein intake and subsequent falls in older men and women: the Framingham Study. J Nutr Health Aging 2011;15:147.
19. Wallace JI, Schwartz RS, LaCroix AZ, et al. Involuntary weight loss in older outpatients: incidence and clinical significance. J Am Geriatr Soc 1995;43:329.
20. Locher JL, Roth DL, Ritchie CS, et al. Body mass index, weight loss, and mortality in community-dwelling older adults. J Gerontol A Biol Sci Med Sci 2007;62:1389–92.
21. Newman AB, Yanez D, Harris T, et al. Weight change in old age and its association with mortality. J Am Geriatr Soc 2001;49:1309.
22. Newman AB, Lee JS, Visser M, et al. Weight change and the conservation of lean mass in old age: the health, aging and body composition study. Am J Clin Nutr 2005;82:872.

23. Janssen I, Baumgartner RN, Ross R, et al. Skeletal muscle cutpoints associated with elevated physical disability risk in older men and women. Am J Epidemiol 2004;159:413.
24. Lee JS, Kritchevsky SB, Tylavsky F, et al. Weight change, weight change intention, and the incidence of mobility limitation in well-functioning community-dwelling older adults. J Gerontol A Biol Sci Med Sci 2005;60:1007.
25. Vanderschueren S, Geens E, Knockaert D, et al. The diagnostic spectrum of unintentional weight loss. Eur J Intern Med 2005;16:160.
26. McMinn J, Steel C, Bowman A. Investigation and management of unintentional weight loss in older adults. BMJ 2011;342:d1732.
27. Stajkovic S, Aitken EM, Holroyd-Leduc J. Unintentional weight loss in older adults. CMAJ 2011;183:443–9.
28. McDermid RC, Stelfox HT, Bagshaw SM. Frailty in the critically ill: a novel concept. Crit Care 2011;15:301.
29. Newman AB, Gottdiener JS, McBurnie MA, et al. Associations of subclinical cardiovascular disease with frailty. J Gerontol A Biol Sci Med Sci 2001;56:M158–66.
30. Gill TM, Baker DI, Gottschalk M, et al. A program to prevent functional decline in physically frail, elderly persons who live at home. N Engl J Med 2002;347:1068.
31. Dickerson RN, Brown RO. Long-term enteral nutrition support and the risk of dehydration. Nutr Clin Pract 2005;20:646.
32. Lipp J, Lord LM, Scholer LH. Techniques and procedures; fluid management in enteral nutrition. Nutr Clin Pract 1999;14:232.
33. Wakefield BJ, Mentes J, Holman JE, et al. Risk factors and outcomes associated with hospital admission for dehydration. Rehabil Nurs 2008;33:233.
34. Agency for Healthcare Research and Quality. Prevention quality indicators overview. Available at: http://www.qualityindicators.ahrq.gov/modules/pqi_overview.aspx. Accessed March 3, 2013.
35. Agency for Healthcare Research and Quality. Prevention quality indicator comparative data: based on the 2009 Nationwide Inpatient Sample (NIS) Version 4.4. Available at: http://www.qualityindicators.ahrq.gov/Downloads/Modules/PQI/V44/Comparative%20Data%20PQI%204.4.pdf. Accessed March 3, 2013.
36. Wakefield BJ, Mentes J, Holman JE, et al. Postadmission dehydration: risk factors, indicators, and outcomes. Rehabil Nurs 2009;34:209.
37. Warren JL, Bacon WE, Harris T, et al. The burden and outcomes associated with dehydration among US elderly, 1991. Am J Public Health 1994;84:1265.
38. Gariballa S, Forster S. Effects of acute-phase response on nutritional status and clinical outcome of hospitalized patients. Nutrition 2006;22:750.
39. Bouillanne O, Hay P, Liabaud B, et al. Evidence that albumin is not a suitable marker of body composition-related nutritional status in elderly patients. Nutrition 2011;27:165.
40. Hiesmayr M. Nutrition risk assessment in the ICU. Curr Opin Clin Nutr Metab Care 2012;15:174.
41. Jensen GL, Wheeler D. A new approach to defining and diagnosing malnutrition in adult critical illness. Curr Opin Crit Care 2012;18:206.
42. Miller KR, Kiraly LN, Lowen CC, et al. "CAN WE FEED?" A mnemonic to merge nutrition and intensive care assessment of the critically ill patient. JPEN J Parenter Enteral Nutr 2011;35:643.
43. Codner PA. Enteral nutrition in the critically ill patient. Surg Clin North Am 2012;92:1485.
44. Dudrick SJ. Nutrition management of geriatric surgical patients. Surg Clin North Am 2011;91:877.

45. Jensen GL. Inflammation as the key interface of the medical and nutrition universes: a provocative examination of the future of clinical nutrition and medicine. JPEN J Parenter Enteral Nutr 2006;30:453.
46. Jensen GL. Inflammation: roles in aging and sarcopenia. JPEN J Parenter Enteral Nutr 2008;32:656.
47. Evans WJ. Skeletal muscle loss: cachexia, sarcopenia, and inactivity. Am J Clin Nutr 2010;91:1123S.
48. Sullivan DH, Sun S, Walls RC. Protein-energy undernutrition among elderly hospitalized patients: a prospective study. JAMA 1999;281:2013.
49. Hiesmayr M, Schindler K, Pernicka E, et al. Decreased food intake is a risk factor for mortality in hospitalized patients: the Nutrition Day survey 2006. Clin Nutr 2009;28:484.
50. Bell L. AACN Practice Alert. Prevention of aspiration. American Association of Critical Care Nurses. Available at: http://www.aacn.org/WD/practice/docs/practicealerts/aacn-aspiration-practice-alert.pdf. Accessed March 3, 2013.
51. Gacouin A, Camus C, Le Tulzo Y, et al. Assessment of peri-extubation pain by visual analogue scale in the adult intensive care unit: a prospective observational study. Intensive Care Med 2004;30:1340.
52. Marik PE. Management of the critically ill geriatric patient. Crit Care Med 2006; 34(Suppl 9):S176.
53. Barrocas A, Geppert C, Durfee SM, et al. ASPEN ethics position paper. Nutr Clin Pract 2010;25:672.
54. Pioneer Network Food and Dining Clinical Standards Task Force. New dining practice standards. Available at: http://www.pioneernetwork.net/Providers/DiningPracticeStandards/. Accessed January 3, 2012.
55. American Society for Parenteral and Enteral Nutrition. Definition of terms, style, and conventions used in ASPEN Board of Directors-approved documents: American Society for Parenteral and Enteral Nutrition. 2012. Available at: http://www.nutritioncare.org/Professional_Resources/Guidelines_and_Standards/Guidelines/2012_Definitions_of_Terms,_Style,_and_Conventions_Used_in_A_S_P_E_N__Board_of_Directors-Approved_Documents/. Accessed June 26, 2013.
56. Joint Commission. Comprehensive accreditation manual for hospitals. Chicago: Joint Commission on Accreditation of Healthcare Organizations; 2007.
57. Chima CS, Dietz-Seher C, Kushner-Benson S. Nutrition risk screening in acute care: a survey of practice. Nutr Clin Pract 2008;23:417–23.
58. Skipper A, Ferguson M, Thompson K, et al. Nutrition screening tools: an analysis of the evidence. JPEN J Parenter Enteral Nutr 2012;36:292.
59. Green SM, Watson R. Nutritional screening and assessment tools for older adults: literature review. J Adv Nurs 2006;54:477.
60. DiMaria-Ghalili RA, Amella E. Assessing nutrition in older adults. Hartford Institute for Geriatric Nursing. Available at: http://consultgerirn.org/uploads/File/trythis/try_this_9.pdf. Accessed March 3, 2013.
61. Cereda E. Mini nutritional assessment. Curr Opin Clin Nutr Metab Care 2012; 15:29.
62. Volkert D, Saeglitz C, Gueldenzoph H, et al. Undiagnosed malnutrition and nutrition-related problems in geriatric patients. J Nutr Health Aging 2010;14:387.
63. Jensen GL, Hsiao PY, Wheeler D. Nutrition screening and assessment. In: Mueller C, editor. The ASPEN Adult nutrition core curriculum. Silver Spring (MD): American Society for Parenteral and Enteral Nutrition; 2012. p. 155.
64. Sabol VK. Nutrition assessment of the critically ill adult. AACN Clin Issues 2004; 15:595.

65. Jensen GL, Hsiao PY, Wheeler D. Adult nutrition assessment tutorial. JPEN J Parenter Enteral Nutr 2012;36:267.
66. National Heart Lung, and Blood Institute Clinical guidelines on the identification, evaluation, and treatment of overweight and obesity in adults: the evidence report. Available at: http://www.nhlbi.nih.gov/guidelines/obesity/ob_gdlns.pdf. Accessed March 3, 2013.
67. White JV, Dwyer JT, Posner BM, et al. Nutrition screening initiative: development and implementation of the public awareness checklist and screening tools. J Am Diet Assoc 1992;92:163.
68. Center for Medicare and Medicaid Services. 2012 Physician quality reporting system measures specification manual for claims and registry: reporting of individual measures. American Medical Association. Available at: http://www.aan.com/globals/axon/assets/9111.pdf. Accessed November 8, 2012.
69. White JV, Guenter P, Jensen G, et al. Consensus statement of the Academy of Nutrition and Dietetics/American Society for Parenteral and Enteral Nutrition: characteristics recommended for the identification and documentation of adult malnutrition (undernutrition). J Acad Nutr Diet 2012;112:730–8.
70. Cherry-Bukowiec JR. Optimizing nutrition therapy to enhance mobility in critically ill patients. Crit Care Nurs Q 2013;36:28–36.
71. Feldblum I, German L, Castel H, et al. Characteristics of undernourished older medical patients and the identification of predictors for undernutrition status. Nutr J 2007;6:37.
72. Norman K, Stobaus N, Gonzalez MC, et al. Hand grip strength: outcome predictor and marker of nutritional status. Clin Nutr 2011;30:135.
73. Guerra RS, Amaral TF. Comparison of hand dynamometers in elderly people. J Nutr Health Aging 2009;13:907.
74. Gross CR, Lindquist RD, Woolley AC, et al. Clinical indicators of dehydration severity in elderly patients. J Emerg Med 1992;10:267.
75. Vivanti A, Harvey K, Ash S, et al. Clinical assessment of dehydration in older people admitted to hospital: what are the strongest indicators? Arch Gerontol Geriatr 2008;47:340.
76. Prins A. Nutritional assessment of the critically ill patient. S Afr J Clin Nutr 2010;23(1):11–8.
77. Jensen GL, Mirtallo J, Compher C, et al. Adult starvation and disease-related malnutrition: a proposal for etiology-based diagnosis in the clinical practice setting from the International Consensus Guideline Committee. JPEN J Parenter Enteral Nutr 2010;34:156.
78. Thomas DR, Cote TR, Lawhorne L, et al. Understanding clinical dehydration and its treatment. J Am Med Dir Assoc 2008;9:292.
79. Mueller C, Zelig R. Nutrition support for older adults. In: Mueller C, editor. The ASPEN adult nutrition support core curriculum. 2nd edition. Silver Springs (MD): American Society for Parenteral and Enteral Nutrition; 2012. p. 620–9.
80. Mueller C. The ASPEN adult nutrition support core curriculum. 2nd edition. Silver Springs (MD): American Society for Parenteral and Enteral Nutrition; 2012.
81. Khalid I, Doshi P, DiGiovine B. Early enteral nutrition and outcomes of critically ill patients treated with vasopressors and mechanical ventilation. Am J Crit Care 2010;19:261.
82. Sullivan D, Lipschitz D. Evaluating and treating nutritional problems in older patients. Clin Geriatr Med 1997;13:753.

83. Woien H, Bjork IT. Nutrition of the critically ill patient and effects of implementing a nutritional support algorithm in ICU. J Clin Nurs 2006;15:168.
84. Heyland DK, Dhaliwal R, Drover JW, et al, Canadian Critical Care Clinical Practice Guidelines Committee. Canadian clinical practice guidelines for nutrition support in mechanically ventilated, critically ill adult patients. JPEN J Parenter Enteral Nutr 2003;27:355.
85. Bankhead R, Boullata J, Brantley S, et al. Enteral nutrition practice recommendations. JPEN J Parenter Enteral Nutr 2009;33:122.
86. Kattelmann KK, Hise M, Russell M, et al. Preliminary evidence for a medical nutrition therapy protocol: enteral feedings for critically ill patients. J Am Diet Assoc 2006;106:1226.
87. Roberts SR, Kennerly DA, Keane D, et al. Nutrition support in the intensive care unit. Adequacy, timeliness, and outcomes. Crit Care Nurse 2003;23:49.
88. Brantley S, Mills ME. Overview of enteral nutrition. In: Mueller C, editor. The ASPEN adult nutrition support core curriculum. 2nd edition. Silver Springs (MD): American Society for Parenteral and Enteral Nutrition; 2012. p. 170–84.
89. Cresci G, Lefton J, Espar D. Enteral formulations. In: Mueller C, editor. The ASPEN adult nutrition support core curriculum. 2nd edition. Silver Springs (MD): American Society for Parenteral and Enteral Nutrition; 2012. p. 185–205.
90. Kump VJ, Gervasio J. Complications of parenteral nutrition. In: Mueller C, editor. The ASPEN adult nutrition support core curriculum. 2nd edition. Silver Springs (MD): American Society for Parenteral and Enteral Nutrition; 2012. p. 284–97.
91. Mirtallo J, Patel M. Overview of parenteral nutrition. In: Mueller C, editor. The ASPEN adult nutrition support core curriculum. 2nd edition. Silver Springs (MD): American Society for Parenteral and Enteral Nutrition; 2012. p. 234–44.
92. Marshall AP, West SH. Enteral feeding in the critically ill: are nursing practices contributing to hypocaloric feeding? Intensive Crit Care Nurs 2006;22:95.
93. Bourgault AM, Ipe L, Weaver J, et al. Development of evidence-based guidelines and critical care nurses ' knowledge of enteral feeding. Crit Care Nurse 2007;27:17.
94. DeLegge MH. Managing gastric residual volumes in the critically ill patient: an update. Curr Opin Clin Nutr Metab Care 2011;14:193.
95. Metheny NA, Mills AC, Stewart BJ. Monitoring for intolerance to gastric tube feedings: a national survey. Am J Crit Care 2012;21:e33.
96. Malone A, Seres D, Lord L. Complications of enteral nutrition. In: Mueller C, editor. The ASPEN adult nutrition support core curriculum. 2nd edition. Silver Springs (MD): American Society for Parenteral and Enteral Nutrition; 2012. p. 218–33.
97. Miller CA, Grossman S, Hindley E, et al. Are enterally fed ICU patients meeting clinical practice guidelines? Nutr Clin Pract 2009;23:642.
98. O'Meara D, Mireles-Cabodevila E, Frame F, et al. Evaluation of delivery of enteral nutrition in critically ill patients receiving mechanical ventilation. Am J Crit Care 2008;17:53.
99. De Jonghe B, Appere-De-Vechi C, Fournier M, et al. A prospective survey of nutritional support practices in intensive care unit patients: what is prescribed? What is delivered? Crit Care Med 2001;29:8.

Infection, Sepsis, and Immune Function in the Older Adult Receiving Critical Care

Camille Lineberry, MSN, ACNP-BC*,
Deborah E. Stein, MSN, ACNP-BC, CCRN

KEYWORDS

- Elderly • Aged • Sepsis • Critical illness • Immune function • Outcomes • ICU

KEY POINTS

- The elderly population (those >65 years old) is projected to increase significantly over the next few decades, leading to increased hospitalizations and utilization of intensive care unit resources for sepsis.
- The elderly have increased vulnerability to developing sepsis due to diminished physiologic reserve, presence of comorbidities, immunosenescence, frequent instrumentation, institutionalization, and clinician underrecognition of infection.
- Infection can vary in severity along a continuum, ranging from mild to severe, including systemic hypotension, tissue hypoperfusion, and organ damage in its most severe form (septic shock).
- Clinical presentation of infection among the elderly is often nonspecific, and can include mental status changes, increased frequency of falls, general malaise, new urinary incontinence, and mild tachypnea. Classic signs, such as fever or leukocytosis, may be absent.
- Diagnostic workup should include blood and body fluid cultures from the suspected infectious source, ideally before antibiotics are initiated, as long as undue delays in treatment do not result. Chest radiography, computed tomography imaging, and echocardiography may be indicated for more in-depth assessment of infected anatomy.
- Cornerstones of sepsis therapy include early recognition; initiation of appropriate, broad-spectrum antibiotics within 1 hour of suspected infection; control of infectious source; and aggressive fluid resuscitation for those with severe sepsis. Vasopressors and other adjunctive therapies may be required for persistent hypotension.
- The elderly are at increased risk for prolonged hospitalization, death, or permanent disability resulting from sepsis. With this in mind, goals of care should be explored with patients and families as soon as possible.

No disclosures to make.
Department of Anesthesiology and Critical Care, Memorial Sloan Kettering Cancer Center, 1275 York Avenue, New York, NY 10065, USA
* Corresponding author.
E-mail address: lineberc@mkscc.org

Crit Care Nurs Clin N Am 26 (2014) 47–60
http://dx.doi.org/10.1016/j.ccell.2013.09.009
0899-5885/14/$ – see front matter © 2014 Elsevier Inc. All rights reserved.

INTRODUCTION

Infections are caused by the invasion of a host's body or tissues by a microorganism. The resultant infectious state may vary in severity, and can progress along a continuum, including the systemic inflammatory response syndrome (SIRS), sepsis, severe sepsis, and septic shock (**Box 1**).[1–6] Sepsis carries a mortality rate of 20% to 50%,[3,7] and approximately 50% of those who develop sepsis require intensive care.[7,8] The incidence of severe sepsis increases with age, most notably in the elderly, with almost 60% of cases occurring in patients 65 years or older.[9] The reasons for increased incidence among the elderly are multifactorial, including diminished physiologic reserve, immunosenescence, presence of comorbidities, subtle clinical presentations, frequent instrumentation, and institutionalization (**Fig. 1**).[1,10–12] Those who survive severe sepsis are more likely to have irreversible organ damage, cognitive impairments, and diminished overall function.[11,13] With an increasingly aging population being admitted to intensive care units (ICUs), it is incumbent on health care practitioners to understand the challenges facing this cohort and how to optimize their management.

EPIDEMIOLOGY

Critical care services for sepsis represent an enormous portion of hospital costs in the United States, much of it consumed by the elderly.[7,10] The elderly are at particular risk for sepsis and severe sepsis, accounting for nearly two-thirds of all patients hospitalized with sepsis in 2008,[13] and, as the population ages, its incidence has been predicted to increase.[9] The National Center for Health Statistics (NCHS) data, published in 2011, confirm the increasing incidence and cost of treating sepsis in hospitalized patients, with hospitalization rates doubling for septicemia or sepsis between 2000 and 2008.[13] According to these data, hospitalizations for patients older than 85 were 30 times higher than for those younger than 65, and there was a fourfold increase in hospitalizations for that age group as compared with patients aged between 65 and 75 years.[13] As the baby boomer population ages, by 2030, the number of octogenarians is expected to double[10] and the population of elderly is expected to exceed that of the young by 2050.[1]

Patients hospitalized with sepsis or septicemia are much more likely to die as compared with those with other diagnoses.[13] According to the NCHS data, 17% of elderly patients with sepsis died, whereas only 2% of those hospitalized for other problems did, and had a 75% longer average length of stay.[13] Angus and colleagues[9] published an article in 2001 documenting that costs of care for patients older than 65 with sepsis represented slightly more than 80% of total costs for severe sepsis, estimated to exceed $16.7 billion. Since then, Lagu and colleagues[14] identified a rapid increase in the number of cases of severe sepsis, with a 71% increase in incidence between 2003 and 2007, and an increase in total hospital costs for all patients ($15.4 billion in 2003 to $24.3 billion in 2007). Given these alarming statistics, understanding of the particular challenges facing the aging population is essential.

To understand the challenges facing the elderly, it is important to have some knowledge of predisposing factors, the most common sites of infection, and causative pathogens to assist with early detection and prompt management of sepsis in this population. Although in almost 50% of cases of sepsis an organism is never identified,[7] when it is identified, gram-negative bacteria are 1.31 times more likely to be the cause of sepsis among patients 65 years or older, with respiratory and genitourinary sources being the most common cause.[7] When gram-positive infections are identified, *Staphylococcus aureus* is most commonly isolated among all age groups, but is more likely to be a drug-resistant phenotype among the elderly.[15] In addition

Box 1
Criteria for systemic inflammatory response syndrome (SIRS), sepsis, severe sepsis, septic shock

SIRS: presence of at least 2 of the following:

Hyperthermia or hypothermia with temperature >38°C or <36°C

Tachycardia (heart rate >90 beats per minute)

Tachypnea (respiratory rate >20 breaths per minute or $Paco_2$ <32 mm Hg)

Leukocytosis or leukopenia (WBC >12,000 cells/mm³, <4000 cells/mm³, or >10% immature forms [bandemia])

Sepsis

SIRS with one of the following:

  Documented infection

  Presence of inflammatory variables, including plasma C-reactive protein more than 2 SD above normal or plasma procalcitonin more than 2 SD above the normal value

Plus some of the following:

  Acute encephalopathy, delirium, or psychosis

  Hyperglycemia (plasma glucose >140 mg/dL) in the absence of diabetes

  Arterial hypoxemia (Pao_2/Fio_2 <300 mm Hg)

  Positive fluid balance >20 mL/kg over 24 hours

  Acute oliguria (urine output <0.5 mL/kg/h for at least 2 hours despite adequate fluid resuscitation)[a]

  Creatinine increase >0.5 mg/dL[a]

  Ileus (absent bowel sounds)[a]

  Hyperbilirubinemia (plasma total bilirubin >4 mg/dL)[a]

  Thrombocytopenia (platelet count <100,000 μL^{-1})[a]

  Coagulation abnormalities (INR >1.5 or aPTT >60 s)[a]

  Disseminated intravascular coagulopathy[a]

  Hypotension (defined as SBP <90 mm Hg, MAP <70, or an SBP decrease >40 mm Hg from baseline)

  Mixed venous oxygen saturation >70%

  Cardiac index >3.5 L/min/m²

  Hyperlactatemia (>3 mmol/L)

  Unexplained metabolic acidosis

  Decreased capillary refill or mottling on physical examination

Severe sepsis

Sepsis with the presence of ≥1 organ dysfunction as evidenced by any of the following:

  Sepsis-induced hypotension

  Hyperlactatemia with lactate above upper limits of laboratory normal

  Persistent oliguria (<0.5 mL/kg/h for >2 hours despite adequate fluid resuscitation)

  Acute lung injury with Pao_2/Fio_2 <250 in the absence of pneumonia source of infection

  Acute lung injury with Pao_2/Fio_2 <200 in the presence of pneumonia source of infection

Creatinine >2 mg/dL

Hyperbilirubinemia (plasma total bilirubin >2 mg/dL)

Transaminitis

Thrombocytopenia (platelet count <100,000 μL^{-1})

Coagulopathy

Septic Shock

Severe sepsis with hypotension that persists despite adequate volume resuscitation necessitating the addition of vasopressors with ongoing evidence of hypoperfusion or organ dysfunction.

Abbreviations: aPTT, activated partial thromboplastin time; F_iO_2, fraction of inspired oxygen; INR, international normalized ratio; MAP, mean arterial blood pressure; $Paco_2$, partial pressure of arterial carbon dioxide; Pao_2, partial pressure of arterial oxygen; SBP, systolic blood pressure; WBC, white blood cell.

   [a] Organ dysfunction criteria.
   Data from Refs.[2,3,15,31]

to methicillin-resistant *Staphylococcus aureus* (MRSA), there is an increased incidence of vancomycin-resistant enterococci (VRE) and extended spectrum β-lactamase (ESBL) *Klebsiella* strains isolated in the elderly.[1] The difference in pathogens is likely related to physiologic changes in the elderly that lead to increased susceptibility to invading microorganisms, presence of chronic comorbid conditions, prior and ongoing instrumentation, such as urinary catheters, prior procedures, increased cumulative exposure to antibiotics, and hospitalization or institutionalization.[1,11,15] Chronic comorbid conditions are present in more than 71% of patients with sepsis, with patients older than 65 being twice as likely to have at least one comorbid condition.[7] The most common comorbid conditions present in elderly patients include coronary artery disease, congestive heart failure, chronic obstructive pulmonary disease, malignancy, and recent surgery.[7,15] With an understanding of causative pathogens

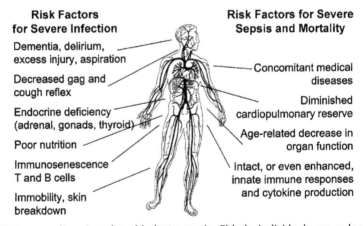

Fig. 1. Factors predisposing the elderly to sepsis. Elderly individuals are vulnerable to the development of severe, life-threatening infections for multifactorial reasons. (*From* Girard TD, Opal SM, Ely EW. Insights into severe sepsis in older patients: from epidemiology to evidence-based management. Clin Infect Dis 2005;40:719–27; with permission.)

and predisposing factors to sepsis in the elderly, we must move on to an understanding of the underlying pathophysiology of sepsis, immune changes in the elderly, and diagnostic and management strategies for this vulnerable population so as to optimize outcomes.

Sepsis Pathophysiology

Sepsis is classically defined as a systemic inflammatory response to a suspected or proven infection, often leading to more lethal forms, including severe sepsis and septic shock, which require treatment in the ICU (see **Box 1**).[5] Severe sepsis is defined as sepsis with the addition of sepsis-induced organ dysfunction or evidence of tissue hypoperfusion.[5] Septic shock is defined as severe sepsis with sepsis-induced hypotension that persists despite adequate fluid resuscitation, and often requires management with vasopressors.[5] The course of sepsis and its outcome depends on a complex interaction of factors. These include characteristics of the infecting organism, including burden of infection; presence of superantigens and other virulence factors; resistance to opsonization and phagocytosis; and susceptibility of the organism to antibiotics.[16] Host responses to infection, including immune, inflammatory, and coagulation responses, impact the course of illness as well.[16] Although the septic state is often thought of as a hyperimmune host response, on closer investigation, it has been found to be associated with a concomitant immunosuppressed state with reduced production of proinflammatory cytokines and unopposed anti-inflammatory mediator release.[17,18] Additionally, cellular dysfunction, as exemplified by neutrophil failure to phagocytize and clear pathogens, plus an abnormal induction of cellular apoptosis, leading to reduced lymphocyte function and amplified neutrophil activity, exacerbate organ injury.[18] The unopposed proinflammatory response leads to further organ dysfunction and critical illness.

The human response to infection comprises a complex interaction among physical barriers to infection, innate and adaptive immune responses, and the coagulation system. In the elderly, particularly those who are critically ill, there are disruptions in all of these systems, leading to increased susceptibility to infection, superinfection, and worse outcomes.[7,11,15]

The Immune System and Sepsis in the Elderly

Immunosenescence

As the human body ages, it undergoes physiologic, biochemical, and hormonal changes that result in a less efficient and dysregulated immune response to pathogens (see **Fig. 1**). This aging process, termed immunosenescence, renders elderly individuals more susceptible to infection, more likely to have a suboptimal response to vaccination, and more likely to experience a chronic, proinflammatory state with a subsequent heightened activation of the systemic inflammatory response system to invading pathogens.[15,19,20] Immunosenescence is incompletely understood, but involves changes to both the innate and adaptive branches of the immune system.

The innate immune system

The innate immune system consists of those immune functions that are inborn, and not subject to modification due to exposure to the environment. Skin and mucosal barriers, macrophages, monocytes, neutrophils, natural killer cells, natural killer T cells, dendritic cells, and the complement system comprise the innate immune system.[20] The innate immune system recognizes the presence of a pathogen, modifies the local environment to contain and eliminate the threat, limits resultant tissue damage, and promotes tissue repair.[17]

Physical barriers to infection include both indigenous microbial flora that exist on the surface of the host, as well as mucosal barriers.[17,21] The presence of symbiotic bacteria preserves normal host defenses by developing and maintaining normal epithelium, particularly within the intestinal tract.[17] This facilitates acute inflammatory responses to injury,[21] and restricts access to potential mucosal binding sites for pathogens.[17] During the treatment course for sepsis, this indigenous flora may be altered by antibiotic therapy, thereby rendering the host susceptible to superinfection with nosocomial organisms, such as *Candida*[17] and *Clostridium difficile*.[11]

In the elderly, specific physiologic changes result in increased susceptibility to infection (see **Fig. 1**). Diminished mucous production and decreased capacity for mucociliary transport, along with impaired swallowing and a diminished cough reflex, increase elderly individuals' risk for contracting pneumonia.[11] Changes in the genitourinary system, including incomplete bladder emptying, vaginal atrophy in postmenopausal women, and benign prostatic hypertrophy in men, predispose the elderly to urinary tract infections (UTIs), one of the most common infections afflicting this population.[7,11,22] Atrophied and hypoperfused skin increases the risk of skin and soft tissue infections, particularly those who are institutionalized, immobilized, or suffering from comorbid conditions, such as diabetes mellitus.[10,11] Changes to the endocrine system, in particular the hypothalamic-pituitary-adrenal axis, result in diminished production of immune-enhancing steroid hormones, also increasing susceptibility to infection among the elderly.[20]

At the molecular level, the innate immune response comprises an initial immune response that is mediated by pathogen pattern-recognition receptors, including toll-like receptors, nucleotide-binding oligomerization domainlike receptors, C-type lectin receptors, and triggering receptors.[16–18] These receptors are expressed on myeloid cells, and interact with invading microorganisms.[16,17] During sepsis, pattern-recognition receptors bind to microbial antigens, initiating intracellular signaling that leads to upregulation of both proinflammatory molecules and anti-inflammatory cytokines.[16] Proinflammatory mediators activate neutrophils and natural killer cell adhesion molecules, which release cytotoxic material that simultaneously kill invading pathogens and create endothelial damage. Endothelial damage, in turn, releases mediators that amplify the inflammatory response systemically, leading to the vasodilatation, systemic hypotension, and multiorgan dysfunction seen in severe sepsis and septic shock.[16,17] At later stages of sepsis, host immunosuppression can result from anergy, lymphopenia, hypothermia, and nosocomial infection, and has been associated with death in patients with sepsis.[11,16,17]

Neutrophil function is decreased in the elderly, with impaired opsonization and phagocytosis of pathogens, as well as diminished chemotaxis, resulting in increased and prolonged inflammation at the site of injury.[20] Increasing age results in reduced precision, efficiency, and competence of nearly every aspect of the innate immune system; additionally, there is a generalized proinflammatory environment created by elevated levels of cytokines that heightens severity of illness in the elderly with sepsis.[19,20]

The adaptive immune system

The adaptive immune system is composed of T-lymphocytes and B-lymphocytes, and is capable of undergoing changes that allow it to identify specific invading pathogens, mount an appropriate response, and "remember" these invaders throughout the life span. The adaptive immune system is mediated by the stimulation of specific humoral-mediated and cell-mediated immune molecules that further amplify the innate immune response.[16] In response to a pathogen, T cells mount the cell-mediated immune response in the form of T helper cells, which produce cytokines that function to direct the immune response, while cytotoxic T cells most commonly express T-cell receptors that recognize specific antigens and produce toxic substances containing enzymes that function to induce apoptosis of pathogen-infected cells. During sepsis, T-cell subgroups are modified, such that helper T cells can be categorized as type 1 helper cells (Th1) or type 2 helper (Th2) cells, each with specific functions.[16] Proinflammatory cytokines are secreted by the Th1 cells, including tumor necrosis factor-α and interleukin (IL)-1β, while the anti-inflammatory cytokines are secreted by the Th2 cells, including IL-4 and IL-10.[16] B cells, on the other hand, produce antibodies and immunoglobulin in response to antigen stimulus; these form complexes that are then recognized by the innate immune system and destroyed.[16,23] The adaptive immune response is contingent on the infecting organism, the burden of infection, and other factors.[16]

Changes to the T-cell–mediated immune response in the elderly include decreased production of naïve T cells by the involuting thymus,[19,24] decreased proliferative response in the presence of infection,[24] decreased production of and response to cytokines,[24] impaired cell-mediated cytotoxicity,[11,15] and lower delayed-type hyper-sensitivity.[11] These changes diminish the elderly individual's ability to fend off infections from new invading organisms, whereas activity against previously recognized pathogens is attenuated by memory T cells that are functionally incompetent, although able to recognize antigens.[19,24] This increases elderly individuals' vulnerability to viral infections, in particular, cytomegalovirus, Epstein-Barr virus, and varicella zoster virus, as well as blunts antibody response to vaccinations.[19]

B-lymphocytes play an important role in antibody-dependent immunity (humoral). Their function is altered in the elderly individual in a number of ways, starting at inception in the bone marrow.[23,25] Fewer B cells are produced in the bone marrow due to deficits in certain genes that facilitate maturation and differentiation of pro–B cell and pre–B cell hematopoietic precursors.[23,26] This diminishes the available naïve B-cell pool capable of presenting antigens to T cells and differentiating to memory cells. Humoral immunity is altered, as memory B cells produce fewer antibodies and immunoglobulin in response to antigen stimulus; some of this attenuation is due to dysfunctional antigen trapping by elements of the innate immune system.[23] Responsiveness to vaccinations, in particular, is decreased because of defects in antibody production at the molecular level within aged B cells.[25]

The Coagulation System

The immune and coagulation systems interact synergistically during sepsis states, to the great detriment of the elderly host, as the presence of proinflammatory cytokines also disrupts the normal modulators of coagulation and inflammation. Lipopolysac-charides, often found on gram-negative bacteria, upregulate endothelial cell tissue factor.[16,17] Tissue factor is also released by activated immune cells and in response to leukocyte-induced endothelial damage, activating the coagulation cascade, which leads to capillary occlusion by microthrombi and end-organ ischemia.[15,16] The coagulation cascade is normally modulated by anticoagulant factors, including protein C, protein S, antithrombin III, and tissue factor-pathway inhibitor; however, these factors are present in much lower levels in the septic state.[16] These anticoagulant factors, particularly activated protein C, in addition to their role in coagulation, augment the immune response by decreasing apoptosis, adhesion of leukocytes, and cytokine production.[18] The elderly have increased levels of coagulation factors, resulting in a prothrombotic state and a heightened response to septic insult.[15] The proinflammatory and procoagulant responses that occur during sepsis not only result from sepsis itself, but from the upregulated release of mediators from hypoperfused, ischemic organs damaged by the shock state further perpetuating this detrimental cycle.[16]

Clinical Presentation

Elderly individuals with sepsis pose a diagnostic challenge to clinicians because they often present with vague, atypical signs and symptoms that also can be found in a wide variety of noninfectious conditions.[1] They are less likely than younger patients to mount a fever or develop leukocytosis in response to infection, although a shift to the left in immature neutrophils is seen.[1,11,15,22] Temperature changes of 1.1°C (2°F) from baseline in the elderly should be considered an infectious response; whereas fevers higher than 38.3°C may signal a life-threatening infection warranting hospitalization.[22]

Nonspecific presenting signs that should alert the clinician to the possibility of infection include new mental status changes, increased falls, general malaise, anorexia, new onset of urinary incontinence, nausea and vomiting, and mild tachypnea (**Box 2**).[11,15,22] Clinicians should be vigilant about looking for evidence of SIRS in elderly individuals presenting with these complaints. A virulent infection leading to severe sepsis and septic shock can easily be overlooked in this population, resulting in a missed opportunity for crucial early interventions and an increase in morbidity and mortality. Although survival from sepsis improves for all age groups with early intervention, the elderly have been shown to particularly benefit from aggressive therapy when it is offered, even though advanced age is an independent risk factor for death from this condition.[1,27,28]

Diagnostic Workup

A diagnostic workup should begin with a high index of suspicion for infection in elderly individuals presenting with vague symptoms, as described in earlier sections. Genitourinary and respiratory tract infections are most common in the elderly (**Box 3**), and should be excluded during history, physical examination, and diagnostic evaluation. Before antibiotics are initiated, whenever feasible, blood (ideally, 2 sets), and body fluid cultures should be obtained from likely sites of infection, including urine, sputum, stool, cerebrospinal fluid, and fluid collections/abscesses.[2] Antibiotics should not be

---

Box 2
Nonspecific signs of infection in the elderly

Mental status changes (somnolence, delirium, coma)

Mild tachypnea

Anorexia

Malaise

Generalized weakness

Increased falls

Unexplained functional decline

Urinary incontinence

Nausea/vomiting

Data from Girard TD, Ely EW. Bacteremia and sepsis in older adults. Clin Geriatr Med 2007;23:633–47, viii; and Mouton CP, Bazaldua OV, Pierce B, et al. Common infections in older adults. Am Fam Physician 2001;63:257–68.

Box 3
Common infections in the elderly
Urinary tract infection
Pneumonia (bacterial or viral)
Influenza
Skin and soft tissue infections
Viral infections
Intra-abdominal infections
Cholecystitis
Diverticulitis
Data from Bender BS. Infectious disease risk in the elderly. Immunol Allergy Clin North Am 2003;23:58, vi.

withheld for more than 45 minutes before obtaining cultures in the setting of severe sepsis and shock states, as delays in initiating antimicrobial therapy, even by hours, have been demonstrated to increase morbidity and mortality.[2] Chest radiographs may be obtained to assess for pneumonia, whereas computed tomography imaging may be required to better assess for suspected pulmonary, intra-abdominal, and soft tissue infections; fluid collections; and abscesses. Echocardiography may be indicated to look for vegetations on the cardiac valves, signaling bacterial endocarditis while also assessing for compromised cardiac function found commonly with severe sepsis and septic shock. Individuals presenting with meningeal symptoms and encephalopathy may require lumbar puncture with cerebrospinal fluid sampling.

Additionally, a basic immune evaluation, including complete blood count with differential should be performed,[11] although nonspecific test values should be interpreted in the context of other diagnostic information as well as the patient's medical history and clinical presentation, as elderly patients do not always develop leukocytosis during active infection.[22] Those who are residents of long-term care facilities or who have frequent contact with the health care system are more likely to be infected with multidrug-resistant organisms, making effective treatment more difficult.[1,22] It also may be difficult to physically obtain culture specimens from patients who are delirious, dehydrated, frail, or unable to comply with positioning requirements because of pain, chronic illness, or osteodegenerative disorders.[1,11,15]

Sepsis Management

Elderly patients are more likely than their younger counterparts to experience a missed diagnosis of infection, progress rapidly to severe sepsis and septic shock, and succumb to their condition.[1] Early, organized, and standardized interventions are crucial to halt progression to septic shock and to limit morbidity and mortality, not the least in the elderly.[26] A landmark trial by Rivers and colleagues[6] in 2001 demonstrated a significant mortality benefit to patients with severe sepsis and septic shock when interventions were provided early and aggressively in the disease state. Shortly thereafter, in 2002, the Surviving Sepsis Campaign (SSC) was launched by the European Society of Intensive Care Medicine, the International Sepsis Forum, and the Society of Critical Care Medicine to standardize sepsis care internationally and thereby reduce mortality through a set of evidence-based guidelines.[4] The SSC was able to find, in

2010, that adoption of these care standards was associated with continuous quality improvement in sepsis care and reduced reported hospital mortality rates among participating international institutions.[4]

It is clear from the data that clinicians must initiate appropriate, aggressive therapy immediately on suspecting infection in all patients with sepsis (**Table 1**). The principle of early intervention is especially important for the elderly, who are at risk for delayed diagnosis and undertreatment, with grave ramifications. Cornerstones of treatment include initiation of appropriately broad-spectrum antibiotic therapy for a suspected pathogen within 1 hour of discovery, source control (removal of suspected infected catheters, devices, and hardware; drainage of abscesses; debridement of wounds), and initiation of aggressive fluid resuscitation with crystalloids in those with severe sepsis and septic shock.[2,10] Initial antibiotic selection for the elderly must take into account the increased likelihood that a gram-negative or multidrug-resistant organism is present, and may include dual therapy for certain organisms.[2] Tailoring antibiotics to a narrower spectrum of coverage can be done later, after culture results and sensitivities are available.[2]

When sepsis-induced tissue hypoperfusion is persistent despite adequate fluid challenge, as evidenced by arterial hypotension, hyperlactatemia, oliguria, or decreased superior vena caval oxygen saturation ($ScvO_2$), vasopressor therapy should be initiated to maintain a mean arterial pressure higher than 65 mm Hg.[2,6] Corticosteroid therapy is recommended in those with systemic shock that is refractory to fluid resuscitation and vasopressor therapy, although low doses should be administered to minimize immunosuppression.[2,15] Additional supportive therapies for conditions associated with severe sepsis and septic shock include red blood cell transfusion for anemia (hemoglobin concentration <7 g/dL)[2]; lung-protective ventilation strategies for those with sepsis-induced acute respiratory distress syndrome[2,15]; minimal use of sedation and daily interruption of sedative infusions with spontaneous weaning trials among intubated, mechanically ventilated patients when clinically appropriate[2,15]; renal replacement therapy for those with life-threatening fluid and electrolyte disturbances from kidney injury[2]; glycemic control to maintain an upper glucose limit of 180 mg/dL or less[2]; enteral feedings, whenever possible, to provide nutrition; and prophylaxis against deep vein thromboses and stress ulcers with daily low-molecular weight heparin and proton pump inhibitors or H2 blockers, respectively.[2,15]

OUTCOMES AND PATIENT PERSPECTIVE

Although advanced age has been noted in most epidemiologic studies as being an independent predictor of death, with age 65 years or older being independently associated with a 2.3 times higher risk of death, severity of illness holds greater prognostic significance.[7,15] Although the elderly have been found to have a greater severity of illness with the presence of shock and renal dysfunction on admission,[29] it has been demonstrated that the elderly do benefit from aggressive interventions.[28] Many elderly have poor premorbid functional status, and are often admitted to acute care institutions from long-term care facilities, with nearly one-third of elderly 80 years or older residing in long-term care facilities.[15] Despite the dearth of data regarding discharge disposition and quality of life among elderly survivors of sepsis and critical illness, there is some evidence demonstrating that quality of life is often maintained among elderly survivors despite the presence of functional decline.[15] To balance this, studies exist that show an increased likelihood for discharge either to long-term care facilities or other hospitals for elderly survivors of sepsis, with lower long-term survival (1–5 years).[7,15,27] The fact that shorter hospital and ICU lengths of stay

Table 1
Key management principles for severe infections in the elderly

Management Principle	Interventions
Early recognition	Nonspecific presenting signs
Appropriate diagnostic tests to identify infectious sources	Complete blood count with differential Blood cultures (at least 2) Urine culture Sputum culture Cerebrospinal fluid culture Tissue cultures
Imaging	Chest radiograph Computed tomography imaging Echocardiography
Timely and appropriate antibiotic administration	Gram-negative infections more common Increased prevalence of multidrug-resistant pathogens Within 1 h of suspecting infection
Control/elimination of suspected infectious sources	Catheters Implanted devices Abscesses Empyema Surgical debridement of necrotic tissue
Early, generous fluid resuscitation for severe sepsis and septic shock	Crystalloids Serial fluid challenges
Vasopressor therapy if fluid resuscitation does not improve septic shock	Persistent hypotension Persistent hyperlactatemia Persistent oliguria Decreased central venous oxygenation
Steroid use for refractory septic shock	Critical illness–related corticosteroid insufficiency Low doses to avoid immunosuppression
Supportive care for organ failures	Lung-protective ventilation strategy Daily interruption of sedative infusions for ventilated patients Spontaneous weaning trials for ventilated patients Renal replacement therapy
Prophylactic regimens	Low molecular weight heparin to prevent venous thromboembolism Proton pump inhibitor or H_2 blocker to prevent gastric stress ulcers
Encourage appropriate vaccinations when recovered	Influenza Pneumococcal
Limit use of catheters	Urinary Vascular

Data from Dellinger RP, Levy MM, Rhodes A, et al. Surviving sepsis campaign: international guidelines for management of severe sepsis and septic shock: 2012. Crit Care Med 2013;41:580–637; and Girard TD, Ely EW. Bacteremia and sepsis in older adults. Clin Geriatr Med 2007;23:633–47, viii.

are associated with the elderly may be a reflection on their overall higher mortality rates, as well as differences in their preferences for aggressive therapy or care limitations imposed by physicians.[7,9,29] A study by Hakim and colleagues[30] for the SUPPORT (Study to Understand Prognoses and Preferences for Outcomes and Risks of

Treatment) investigators, found that the most important predictor of the timing of do-not-resuscitate (DNR) orders was patient preference, although only 52% of patients who preferred to be DNR actually had such orders in place. Furthermore, DNR orders were written more quickly for patients 75 years or older regardless of prognosis.[30] As such, it is imperative that goals of care and prognosis be discussed with patients and their families as early as feasible, and no later than 72 hours after ICU admission.[2] Furthermore, these preferences should be incorporated into treatment and end-of-life care planning using palliative care principles and services as appropriate and when available.[2]

SUMMARY

The elderly are a group at significant risk for increased morbidity and mortality from sepsis. A constellation of factors, including diminished physiologic reserve, immunosenescence, comorbid illness, institutionalization, frequent instrumentation, and decreased access to care makes them particularly vulnerable to developing life-threatening infections. Their clinical presentation is often atypical, leading to missed diagnoses and delays in appropriate treatment, contributing to increased morbidity in this population. Clinicians should therefore have heightened awareness of the potential for sepsis when evaluating elderly patients with vague, nonspecific complaints, with particular attention to changes in mental status. Those who develop severe sepsis and septic shock should be treated according to standardized protocols set forth in the Surviving Sepsis Campaign, with an emphasis on early, aggressive antibiotic therapy, source control, and fluid resuscitation, so as to reduce overall morbidity and mortality.

The elderly presently consume a disproportionate share of critical care resources and health care expenditures, and this is projected to increase over the next decades. Although they comprise a majority within the septic cohort, are more likely to die from sepsis, and have been shown to respond well to aggressive intervention, they are frequently underrepresented and often entirely excluded from clinical trials focused on management of this disease. Indeed, whereas age has been found to be an independent predictor of mortality, it has been shown that the elderly benefit from early, aggressive therapy when offered, and, thus, advanced age should not preclude ICU admission. However, although every effort should be made to provide aggressive care, it should be understood that the elderly are more likely to develop permanent disabilities and organ dysfunction from sepsis and ICU admission and may not return to baseline function. Additionally, they may require long-term institutionalization and face a higher risk of 5-year mortality. With this in mind, efforts should be made to determine patients' and families' preferences for aggressiveness of medical care and expectations about quality of life following discharge, and to institute DNR orders when appropriate.

REFERENCES

1. Nasa P, Juneja D, Singh P. Severe sepsis and septic shock in the elderly: an overview. World J Crit Care Med 2012;1:23–30.
2. Dellinger RP, Levy MM, Rhodes A, et al. Surviving sepsis campaign: international guidelines for management of severe sepsis and septic shock: 2012. Crit Care Med 2013;41:580–637.
3. Kleinpell RM, Graves BT, Ackerman MH. Incidence, pathogenesis, and management of sepsis: an overview. AACN Adv Crit Care 2006;17:385–93.

4. Levy MM, Dellinger RP, Townsend SR, et al. The Surviving Sepsis Campaign: results of an international guideline-based performance improvement program targeting severe sepsis. Crit Care Med 2010;38:367–74.
5. Levy MM, Fink MP, Marshall JC, et al. 2001 SCCM/ESICM/ACCP/ATS/SIS international sepsis definitions conference. Crit Care Med 2003;31:1250–6.
6. Rivers E, Nguyen B, Havstad S, et al. Early goal-directed therapy in the treatment of severe sepsis and septic shock. N Engl J Med 2001;345:1368–77.
7. Martin GS, Mannino DM, Moss M. The effect of age on the development and outcome of adult sepsis. Crit Care Med 2006;34:15–21.
8. Angus DC, Kelley MA, Schmitz RJ, et al. Caring for the critically ill patient. Current and projected workforce requirements for care of the critically ill and patients with pulmonary disease: can we meet the requirements of an aging population? JAMA 2000;284:2762–70.
9. Angus DC, Linde-Zwirble WT, Lidicker J, et al. Epidemiology of severe sepsis in the United States: analysis of incidence, outcome, and associated costs of care. Crit Care Med 2001;29:1303–10.
10. Girard TD, Opal SM, Ely EW. Insights into severe sepsis in older patients: from epidemiology to evidence-based management. Clin Infect Dis 2005;40:719–27.
11. Bender BS. Infectious disease risk in the elderly. Immunol Allergy Clin North Am 2003;23:57–64, vi.
12. De Gaudio AR, Rinaldi S, Chelazzi C, et al. Pathophysiology of sepsis in the elderly: clinical impact and therapeutic considerations. Curr Drug Targets 2009;10:60–70.
13. Hall MJ, Williams SM, DeFrances CJ, et al. Inpatient care for septicemia or sepsis: a challenge for patients and hospitals. NCHS Data Brief 2011;(62):1–8.
14. Lagu T, Rothberg MB, Shieh MS, et al. Hospitalizations, costs, and outcomes of severe sepsis in the United States 2003 to 2007. Crit Care Med 2012;40:754–61.
15. Girard TD, Ely EW. Bacteremia and sepsis in older adults. Clin Geriatr Med 2007; 23:633–47, viii.
16. Russell JA. Management of sepsis. N Engl J Med 2006;355:1699–713.
17. Marshall JC, Charbonney E, Gonzalez PD. The immune system in critical illness. Clin Chest Med 2008;29:605–16, vii.
18. Remick DG. Pathophysiology of sepsis. Am J Pathol 2007;170:1435–44.
19. McElhaney JE, Effros RB. Immunosenescence: what does it mean to health outcomes in older adults? Curr Opin Immunol 2009;21:418–24.
20. Shaw AC, Joshi S, Greenwood H, et al. Aging of the innate immune system. Curr Opin Immunol 2010;22:507–13.
21. Plowden J, Renshaw-Hoelscher M, Engleman C, et al. Innate immunity in aging: impact on macrophage function. Aging Cell 2004;3:161–7.
22. Mouton CP, Bazaldua OV, Pierce B, et al. Common infections in older adults. Am Fam Physician 2001;63:257–68.
23. Cancro MP, Hao Y, Scholz JL, et al. B cells and aging: molecules and mechanisms. Trends Immunol 2009;30:313–8.
24. Weng NP. Aging of the immune system: how much can the adaptive immune system adapt? Immunity 2006;24:495–9.
25. Frasca D, Blomberg BB. Effects of aging on B cell function. Curr Opin Immunol 2009;21:425–30.
26. Geiger H, Rudolph KL. Aging in the lympho-hematopoietic stem cell compartment. Trends Immunol 2009;30:360–5.
27. Rosenthal GE, Kaboli PJ, Barnett MJ, et al. Age and the risk of in-hospital death: insights from a multihospital study of intensive care patients. J Am Geriatr Soc 2002;50:1205–12.

28. El Solh AA, Akinnusi ME, Alsawalha LN, et al. Outcome of septic shock in older adults after implementation of the sepsis "bundle". J Am Geriatr Soc 2008;56: 272–8.

29. Vosylius S, Sipylaite J, Ivaskevicius J. Determinants of outcome in elderly patients admitted to the intensive care unit. Age Ageing 2005;34:157–62.

30. Hakim RB, Teno JM, Harrell FE Jr, et al. Factors associated with do-not-resuscitate orders: patients' preferences, prognoses, and physicians' judgments. SUPPORT Investigators. Study to understand prognoses and preferences for outcomes and risks of treatment. Ann Intern Med 1996;125:284–93.

31. Levy MM, Fink MP, Marshall JC, et al. 2001 SCCM/ESICM/ACCP/ATS/SIS international sepsis definitions conference. Intensive Care Med 2003;29:530–8.

Cardiovascular Issues in Older Adults

Leslie L. Davis, PhD, RN, ANP-BC, FAANP, FAHA

KEYWORDS

- Cardiovascular • Critical care • Elderly • Nursing care • Heart failure
- Myocardial infarction • Hypertension

KEY POINTS

- Nurses need to assess older adults carefully because signs and symptoms are more likely to be more subtle or atypical in elders as compared with younger patients.
- Nurses should monitor elderly patients for side effects of medications, especially if underlying kidney or liver impairment exists.
- Patients in their advanced years have the most benefit to gain with use of guideline-directed medical therapy.

INTRODUCTION

Patients who are 65 years and older make up nearly half of intensive care unit (ICU) admissions and approximately 60% of the ICU hospital days in the United States.[1] Cardiovascular (CV) conditions are commonly the first or second diagnosis on admission to the ICU. Furthermore, even if an elderly patient is not admitted for a CV condition, the physiologic stress of any acute illness challenges the heart, often producing structural or functional compromise. For example, acute ischemia or dysrhythmias may be the primary condition *or* a consequence of an initial physiologic insult.

Critically ill elders are a physiologically diverse group. Their heterogeneity sometimes makes it difficult to separate physiologic aging from the pathology of disease.[2] Moreover, as individuals age, comorbid conditions become more prevalent, making diagnosis and treatment of acute illnesses more challenging. In addition, medications used to treat underlying conditions further predispose elders to physiologic compromise during an acute illness.

Disclosures: No disclosures to report.
School of Nursing, University of North Carolina, 308 Moore Building, PO Box 26170, Greensboro, NC 27402-6170, USA
E-mail address: LLDavis4@uncg.edu

Crit Care Nurs Clin N Am 26 (2014) 61–89
http://dx.doi.org/10.1016/j.ccell.2013.10.004
0899-5885/14/$ – see front matter © 2014 Elsevier Inc. All rights reserved.

The most common CV conditions that nurses encounter when caring for critically ill elders include hypertension (HTN), acute coronary syndromes (ACS), heart failure (HF), conduction disorders (eg, atrial fibrillation [AF]), and valvular heart disease. This article focuses primarily on the first 3 conditions because they have the highest prevalence in the elderly population. In all the conditions, however, there are common threads among elderly patients hospitalized in the ICU. First, cognitive decline among some elderly patients makes history taking challenging for health care providers, regardless of the presenting condition. Second, because symptoms in elders are often subtle, it is frequently difficult to tease out new symptoms from symptoms related to an acute exacerbation of a chronic CV condition. In addition, some elders have underlying conditions that have not been formally diagnosed or treated in the past, making interpretation of diagnostic testing difficult because baseline comparisons are unavailable. Finally, as individuals age, they experience decline in kidney and liver function, which influences laboratory findings (eg, cardiac biomarkers, such as troponin or brain natriuretic peptide values) and the way that individuals are treated medically.

PHYSIOLOGIC CHANGES TO THE HEART

Age-related changes to the CV system affect both the physiologic functioning of the heart *and* the way elderly individuals respond to medical therapy to treat CV conditions. These changes occur progressively over time; however, some individuals decline more rapidly than others.[1] Some of the physiologic changes are related to chronologic age itself, whereas others are related to lifestyle. As a result of these physiologic changes, over time, there are decreases in maximal heart rate (HR), ejection fraction (EF), and cardiac output (CO). **Table 1** gives a summary of age-related physiologic changes to the heart.[1–4]

Hypertension

Burden of the condition
Approximately two-thirds of adults age 65 and older have HTN, and this figure increases to nearly 80% among those 75 and older. This is primarily because as individuals age, systolic blood pressure (SBP) tends to steadily increase, regardless of whether the individuals are being treated for HTN.[5] Diastolic blood pressure (DBP), on the other hand, peaks in the fourth or fifth decade of life, then steadily decreases over time.[5] Therefore, when considering baseline blood pressure (BP) readings outside the hospital, it is common for most elders to have isolated systolic HTN.[4]

Unfortunately, only about three-fourths (71%) of adults age 65 and older are aware that they have the HTN.[6] Furthermore, among those diagnosed with HTN, only about 69% receive treatment and fewer than half (48.8%) reach BP treatment goals.[6] Control rates are worse for elders age 80 and older, with only 38% of men and 23% of women meeting BP treatment goals.[6] For these reasons, elders are more likely to have complications related to uncontrolled HTN.

Hypertension crisis
One of the complications of uncontrolled HTN is an HTN crisis, which occurs in approximately 1% to 2% of those with HTN.[7] Although this percentage is low compared with the high prevalence of HTN in elders, the consequences of having an HTN crisis can be devastating. Formerly referred to as malignant HTN or accelerated HTN, currently an HTN crisis may be classified as HTN urgency or HTN emergency. Distinguishing between an urgent and an emergent HTN crisis is not based solely on BP measurement; instead, it is based on whether end-organ damage exists.[7] Specifically, HTN urgency is defined as an abrupt rise in BP *without* signs of end-organ

Table 1
Physiologic changes to the heart related to aging

Physiologic Change	Physiologic Mechanism	Consequences
Gradual loss of physiologic reserve	• Physiologic stress (eg, blood loss, hypoxia, sepsis, volume depletion). • Vasoconstriction and sodium/water retention in the short term ↑ CO. • Vasoconstriction persists to ↑ afterload. Eventually heart fails to overcome ↑ afterload.	• More vulnerable to disease. • LV volume ↑ over time → fluid in alveoli; pulmonary edema develops. • Maximum oxygen uptake ↓; hypoxemia occurs resulting in poor tissue/cellular perfusion. • CV function ↓. • Kidney function ↓. • Elasticity of skin and lungs ↓.
Decreased response to sympathetic stimulation	• Overall, declining receptor function and autonomic dysregulation. • Activity of SNS ↑ due to receptor dysfunction. • Activity of beta-receptor function ↓. • Baroreceptor reflex response ↓.	• Orthostatic hypotension may result. • Less likely to ↑ HR to compensate for ↓ CO. • Need to ↑ preload or ventricular filling and stroke volume to compensate. • If hypovolemia exists, more likely to decompensate.
Increased stiffness of heart and blood vessels	• Arteriosclerotic process creates stiff arterial and ventricular walls. • Stiff ventricular walls become dependent on atrial contraction (atrial kick). • Atrial dilatation occurs as ventricles become stiff.	• Atrial kick needed for diastolic filling. • Atrial kick lost if in atrial fibrillation (↓ diastolic filling time). • Increased resistance to ventricular ejection due to ↓ ventricular compliance. • Diastolic dysfunction results.
Increased incidence of hypertension	• Arterial distensibility ↓, especially large vessels.	• More likely to have isolated systolic HTN. • Afterload ↑; more likely to develop LVH. • Progressive kidney dysfunction.
Increased incidence of ischemic heart disease	• Longer exposure to risk factors and becoming less active. • More likely to ↑ HR with physiologic stress to maintain CO; exacerbates ischemia.	• Rate-related ischemia more common. • Symptoms may be atypical or absent.
Increased incidence of heart failure	• Progressive ↓ of cardiac myocytes. • Progressive ↑ in myocardial collagen. • Arterial distensibility ↓ resulting in ↓ CO. • CO less responsive to ↑ HR; have to ↑ preload to maintain (or ↑) CO.	• Resting CO more likely to be maintained. • Acute illness ↑ dysfunction. • More likely to have impaired relaxation (diastolic dysfunction). • More dependent on preload. • Minor changes in fluid status may cause decompensation.

(continued on next page)

Table 1 (continued)		
Physiologic Change	**Physiologic Mechanism**	**Consequences**
Increased incidence of dysrhythmias	• Autonomic tissue replaced by connective tissue and fat. • Fibrosis creates conduction abnormalities through intranodal tract and bundle of His.	• May lead to sick sinus syndrome, atrial dysrhythmias, or bundle branch blocks. • Atrial dysrhythmias most common. • Sudden loss of atrial kick with atrial dysrhythmia may cause angina, HF, and/or ↓ BP.

Abbreviations: BP, blood pressure; CO, cardiac output; CV, cardiovascular; HF, heart failure; HR, heart rate; HTN, hypertension; LV, left ventricular; LVH, left ventricular hypertrophy; SNS, sympathetic nervous system; ↑, increase; ↓, decrease.
   Data from Refs.[1–4]

damage. HTN urgency typically occurs when the DBP is 120 mm Hg or greater. Patients diagnosed with HTN urgency need to have their BP controlled within 24 hours to several days.[7] This group of patients may be treated with oral medications on an outpatient basis.

In contrast, an HTN emergency is defined as an abrupt rise in BP that is associated with CV, kidney, or central nervous system end-organ damage.[7] Individuals diagnosed with an HTN emergency require immediate medical attention because of the life-threatening nature of the situation and the increased likelihood of end-organ damage (encephalopathy, acute aortic dissection, stroke, ACS, acute pulmonary edema, and kidney failure). These patients are typically admitted to the ICU for treatment. Thus, the remainder of this section related to HTN crisis, focuses on this group of critically ill elders.

Cause of an HTN crisis

Most patients who have an HTN crisis have uncontrolled HTN as their baseline, but many of them have never been formally diagnosed with high BP. Other common risk factors include kidney disease (renal artery stenosis, glomerulonephritis, or renal cell carcinoma), endocrine disorders (diabetes, Cushing syndrome, primary hyperaldosterism, pheochromocytoma), drugs (cocaine, sympathomimetics, abrupt withdrawal of some antihypertensive agents), central nervous system disorders (head or spinal cord injury, cerebral infarction or hemorrhage, brain tumor), and postoperative pain or complications.[7] However, the mechanisms that trigger an HTN crisis on a particular day are not completely understood. Normally at baseline, even with fluctuations in BP throughout the day, an individual's compensatory mechanisms allow for a relatively constant perfusion to vital organs.[8] Yet, in the case of an HTN crisis, an initial insult serves as the stimulus to abruptly increase BP.[7] The arterioles sense this sharp increase in BP and signal to the vascular endothelium to release nitric oxide (a vasodilator) as a means to compensate.[7] In addition, the arterial smooth muscle contracts to reduce the rise in BP. Over time, however, the endothelium is unable to release enough nitric oxide to buffer the severe and sudden rise in BP. Compensatory mechanisms fail as a result of prolonged arterial smooth muscle contraction, a gradual increase in endothelial dysfunction, and an inability to release more nitric oxide, resulting in rapid and progressive decompensation of vital organ function.[7,8] One of the most serious consequences of a HTN emergency is cerebral edema and microhemorrhages that result from the elevated pressure. These are due to the inability of the brain's autoregulation to tolerate sudden severe changes in BP (increases or decreases). Thus, neurologic deficits occur due to the vasodilation, edema, and increased intracranial pressure (ICP). Interestingly, some patients with a long history of HTN are able to tolerate the acute increase in mean arterial pressure (MAP) without increasing cerebral perfusion, thereby avoiding an increase in ICP.

Obtaining accurate BP readings in elders

It is imperative that nurses measure BP correctly for all patients in the ICU, especially those with suspected HTN emergencies. Nurses need to consider 3 things that affect BP readings: (1) physiologic differences in elders that may influence manual or noninvasive readings; (2) differences in values obtained by noninvasive and invasive methods; and (3) differences between SBP versus MAP readings. Nurses should know that it is common for elderly patients to have an ausculatory gap, a period during manual BP measurement when the true SBP fades away, then recurs at a lower pressure point.[4] This is usually associated with vascular disease caused by long-standing HTN. Thus, when taking manual BP readings, the cuff needs to be inflated high enough to capture the true starting point of the SBP, or otherwise the reading may be falsely low. Additionally, some elders have pseudohypertension, a falsely elevated SBP resulting from markedly sclerotic arteries that will not collapse as the BP cuff is inflated.[4] To assess for this abnormality, the nurse should palpate the pulse distal to the location of the BP cuff during measurement.[4] If the pulse remains palpable, despite having the BP cuff inflated above the SBP, the nurse should suspect pseudohypertension. In this case, only direct measurement of BP (eg, via an arterial line) will reveal an accurate BP.[4]

Nurses also need to be aware of the differences between noninvasive blood pressure (NIBP) readings and invasive arterial pressure readings, which are made when patients experience extremes in BP.[9] Specifically, when a patient is hypotensive, the NIBP runs higher than invasive BP for SBP readings. When a patient is hypertensive, the NIBP runs lower than with the invasive method. Thus, during hypotensive or hypertensive episodes, the NIBP may not capture the full extent of deviation. Furthermore, NIBP systolic readings are not as sensitive as intra-arterial readings in assessing a patient's risk of developing acute kidney injury. Lehman and colleagues[9] advise that if NIBP readings are used, nurses should avoid hypoperfusion in those at risk for acute kidney injury; parameters for the lower limit of the SBP should be higher than the usual threshold of lower than 90 mm Hg. These findings, however, do not mean that an invasive method should be used to obtain BP in every patient in the ICU, just that these differences should be considered.

Regardless of which method is used to obtain the BP, the MAP is a more consistent metric than SBP to use to guide therapy in the ICU.[9] The MAP is the "true driving pressure" for peripheral blood flow.[9] Unfortunately, nursing practice has been slow to adopt use of MAP, especially when NIBP methods are used. Generally, the upper threshold for MAP is between 60 and 65 mm Hg, but goals may be individualized by the medical team based on comorbid conditions.[9]

Evaluation of patients with HTN emergencies

In addition to obtaining accurate BP readings, it is vital to conduct a thorough history and physical examination as part of the admission assessment of a patient with an HTN emergency. If the patient is unable to provide the information, the nurse should ask whether someone close to the patient (a family member, caregiver, partner) is available to provide the information. Assessment of medical history should include history of antihypertensive treatment, including adherence to the regimen, illicit drug use, symptoms of other CV conditions (eg, HF, angina, aortic dissection), symptoms of neurologic deficits (eg, nausea, vomiting, headache, mental status changes, weakness, blurred vision), and symptoms of kidney disease (eg, hematuria or oliguria). In addition, ascertaining whether the patient has a history of thyroid disease, Cushing syndrome, systemic lupus, or systemic sclerosis is helpful in determining potential causes.

A focused physical examination should include a CV and neurologic assessment. As part of the CV examination, BP should be measured in both arms, to check for differences. In addition, the nurse should assess for absent or delayed peripheral pulses (to rule out dissection), auscultate heart and lung sounds (extra heart sounds, such as an S_3, or adventitious lung sounds, such as rales, to rule out pulmonary edema), and check the mental status of the patient as part of neurologic checks (to rule out cerebral hypoperfusion). A fundoscopic examination should also be done by the medical team to assess for soft exudates, hemorrhages, and papilledema. Diagnostic tests should include a 12-lead electrocardiogram (ECG), a chest radiograph, a brain computed tomography scan, and laboratory assessments, including urinalysis, electrolytes with a serum creatinine, complete blood count, cardiac enzymes (especially if acute ischemia is suspected), and BNP, especially if acute HF is suspected.

Treatment of HTN crises

Treatment for an HTN crisis is challenging because there is a lack of evidence-based guidelines for clinical care, especially for elders. However, there are general treatment recommendations for patients with an HTN emergency. The first order of treatment, in addition to determining whether the HTN crisis is an emergent crisis or an urgent crisis, is to address and control any acute precipitating causes (eg, anxiety, pain, hypoxia, hypercapnia, or hypoglycemia).[10] The patient also should be admitted to the ICU and given parenteral medications to reverse end-organ damage related to an HTN emergency.[10] During this time, intra-arterial BP monitoring is required when using certain intravenous (IV) medications, to obtain the most accurate readings.[10]

When treating a patient with an HTN emergency, a critical point to remember is that the BP does not need to be corrected urgently. Too rapid reduction of BP can result in serious ischemia, cortical blindness, hemiplegia, acute myocardial infarction (MI), and/ or acute kidney failure, especially with elders who have long-standing HTN.[10] Instead, allowing a patient's autoregulation to adapt to the clinical situation by decreasing the BP more slowly results in better outcomes. The treatment goal is to restore normal perfusion pressure to the vital organs, not to reach the "normal" target BP goal established for outpatients.[8]

Initially BP measurements should be assessed every 5 to 10 minutes (after the first measurement is obtained).[10] A good rule of thumb is that the MAP should be lowered over a period of 2 to 6 hours after the time of presentation, but not by more than 25% of the initial value at presentation.[7] This should translate to about a 10% decrease in the first hour, with another 15% decrease over the next 2 to 3 hours.[7] To accomplish this, medications need to be effective within the first hour after diagnosis.[10] An exception to this rule is patients experiencing an aortic dissection. In this case, the target SBP should be 120 mm Hg within the first 20 minutes; then an SBP between 100 and 120 mm Hg should be maintained.[7] To do so, medications need to be effective within the first 10 minutes after diagnosis.[10] In the case of an aortic dissection, because SBP is being lowered more rapidly than in other HTN emergencies, the nurse should monitor the patient closely for signs and symptoms of cerebral hypoperfusion (eg, nausea, headache, confusion, psychomotor slowing, or agitation). **Table 2** provides a summary of steps in the nursing care of patients with HTN emergencies, including specific BP goals for various clinical situations.

Table 2
Nursing care for hypertensive emergencies

General BP goals: Lower MAP within 2–6 h of presentation, no more than 25% of the initial value at presentation. BP should be decreased ~10% in the first hour, then ~15%, gradually over 2–3 h. Exception: aortic dissection (see below).

Consequences of HTN Emergency	Signs and Symptoms	Implications for Treatment
Encephalopathy	• Symptoms of cerebral edema or hypoperfusion: nausea/vomiting, headache, psycho-motor agitation or slowing, visual changes, stupor, seizures, delirium, or papilledema. • Rare focal neurologic deficits include: paralysis, paresthesias, loss of muscle control/tone in a specific part of the body; voice, vision, or hearing loss.	• Target BP: MAP lowered by maximum 20% or to DBP 100–110 mm Hg within the first hour, then gradual reduction in BP to "normal" range over 48–72 h. • Medications of choice: intravenous sodium nitroprusside or labetalol.
Ischemic stroke or intracerebral hemorrhage	• Focal neurologic deficits (as above) suggest ischemic stroke or intracerebral hemorrhage.	• Target BP for ischemic stroke: MAP lowered no more than 15%–25%, DBP should not be <100–110 mm Hg in first 24 h. Some thrombolytic protocols may allow for more aggressive BP goals. • Target BP for ischemic stroke post-tPA: SBP <180 mm Hg or DBP <110 mm Hg. • Target BP for intracerebral hemorrhage: MAP lowered by 20%–25%.
Aortic dissection	• Abrupt onset of ripping or tearing sensation in the chest, back, or both. • May mimic symptoms of acute myocardial ischemia, acute HF, stroke, musculoskeletal or pleuritic pain, or an acute abdomen. • Need to monitor for neurologic signs/symptoms of cerebral hypoperfusion, especially if BP is reduced too fast.	• Target BP: SBP 120 mm Hg after 20 min, then maintain at 100–120 mm Hg. • Medications of choice: combination of nitroprusside and beta-blocker (esmolol or labetalol). • Administer beta-blocker before nitroprusside because of the rapid onset of action to avoid reflex tachycardia that could worsen dissection.
Acute coronary syndrome, including acute MI	• Ischemic symptoms, such as pain or pressure in the jaw, neck, chest, arm, or back. Atypical symptoms may include dyspnea at rest or exertion, diaphoresis, and/or nausea. • Some elders have silent ischemia.	• Target BP: MAP 60–100 mm Hg. • Medications of choice: nitrates (nitroglycerin) and beta-blockers. • Avoid enalaprilat, nicardipine, or hyralazine (may induce reflex tachycardia and ↑ workload of heart).

(continued on next page)

Table 2 (continued)		
LV failure	• Acute pulmonary edema may be the cause or consequence of HTN crisis. • ↑ shortness of breath, hypoxia, pulmonary edema on examination or x-ray.	• Target BP: MAP 60–100 mm Hg. • Medications of choice: sodium nitroprusside, nitroglycerin, IV enalaprilat, loop diuretics. Avoid labetalol, esmolol, and nicardipine in acute HF.
Acute renal insufficiency	• Proteinuria, elevated serum creatinine, hypokalemic metabolic alkalosis, and microangiopathic hemolytic anemia. • Level of kidney failure influenced by baseline kidney function.	• Target BP: MAP lowered by 20%–25%. • Medication of choice: fenoldopam. • Avoid use of sodium nitroprusside in acute renal insufficiency.
Postop HTN	• Significantly elevated BP within 2 h after surgery. • Common causes: sympathetic activation and adrenergic surge postop, urinary retention, discontinuing anti-HTN agents preop.	• Target BP: MAP lowered by 20%–25%. • Medication of choice: nicardipine, sodium nitroprusside, esmolol, or labetalol. • Caution: nicardipine may cause perioperative bleeding.

Abbreviations: BP, blood pressure; DBP, diastolic blood pressure; HF, heart failure; HTN, hypertension; IV, intravenous; LV, left ventricular; MAP, mean arterial pressure; Postop, postoperative; Preop, preoperative; SBP, systolic blood pressure; tPA, tissue plasminogen activator; ↑, increase.
  Data from Refs.[7,8,10,11]

Treatment for HTN emergencies

In addition to avoiding an abrupt reduction in BP, nurses treating elders with HTN emergencies should start with lower doses of medications, assess for side effects frequently, and be aware that many elders are admitted with a fluid volume deficit. Volume depletion on arrival at the ICU is likely to be due to pressure-induced natriuresis, which may be the patient's baseline status if the patient is dehydrated, especially in the summer months.[4,11] Thus, unless there are clear signs of fluid overload, administration of loop diuretics should be avoided in elders presenting with an HTN emergency. In fact, in some cases of volume depletion, patients may need volume expansion.

There are different routes of administration for medications to treat HTN emergencies. The IV route is most common because of the relatively short half-life, making these agents easier to titrate, more flexible to use, more likely to have a rapid onset of action, and more likely to have a shorter duration.[9] It is important to note that sublingual administration of phentolamine, clonidine, diazoxide, or nifedipine is *contraindicated* due to the likelihood of severe hypotension with use.[9]

Most IV agents require intra-arterial BP monitoring and continuous ECG monitoring during the acute phase of an HTN emergency to assess for changes in perfusion status.[9] Some agents are preferred over others, depending on the patient's condition(s) at the time of presentation (eg, cerebral edema, aortic dissection, acute ischemic or hemorrhagic stroke, ACS, acute HF, or acute kidney failure, or if a patient is in the acute postoperative setting). Once the BP is stabilized with IV medications, a conversion to oral therapy typically occurs within 6 to 12 hours.[6] **Table 3** provides information on the most common medications used to treat HTN emergencies.

Table 3
Common medications used to treat hypertensive emergencies

Medication/Indication	Action	Dosing Information	Nursing Implications (in Addition to Monitoring for Hypotension)
Sodium nitroprusside Most HTN emergencies, except acute HF.	Vasodilator, arterial and venous. ↓ preload and ↓↓ afterload. (No effect on cardiac output.) ↓ pulmonary capillary wedge pressure and central venous pressure (by ↓ preload). ↓ systemic vascular resistance (↓ afterload).	0.25–10 μg/kg/min IV infusion; maximum dose for 10 min only. Onset of action: seconds to 2 min. Duration: 1–3 min. Should start low and assess frequently.	Side effects: nausea/vomiting/↑ ICP, may develop cyanide toxicity (especially in those with kidney or liver impairment), acidosis, coronary steal syndrome (can shunt blood from diseased vessels to well-perfused vessels). Watch for: cerebral hypoperfusion (due to ↑ ICP), ↓ coronary perfusion, and ototoxicity. Cautious use: elders and those with kidney impairment. May ↓ BP too rapidly.
Nitroglycerin Most HTN emergencies, especially acute coronary ischemia or post-CABG. Helpful if given in combination with diuretics, especially for acute pulmonary edema.	Vasodilator (venous dilation with lower doses; arterial dilation too with higher doses). Smooth muscle vasodilation via nitric oxide. ↓↓ preload and ↓ afterload. (No effect on cardiac output.)	5–100 μg/min IV infusion. Onset of action: 2–5 min. Duration: 5–10 min. Titrate to desired response.	Administer in glass containers and use special tubing. Side effects: headache, reflex tachycardia, vomiting, flushing. Tolerance may develop if administered continuously for 24–48 h. Contraindications: cerebral hemorrhage (↑ ICP) and closed-angle glaucoma.
Fenoldopam Most hypertensive emergencies, especially acute kidney impairment or acute HF.	Vasodilator, arterial. Selective peripheral dopamine-receptor agonist. ↑ perfusion to kidneys. ↓ afterload; ↑ cardiac output; no effect on preload.	0.1–0.6 μg/kg/min IV infusion; increments must not exceed 0.1 μg/kg/min at 20-min intervals. Maximum dose: 1.7 μg/kg/min. Onset of action: 4–15 min. Duration: 30 min–4 h.	May administer without intra-arterial BP monitoring. May withdraw without tapering. Side effects: headache (common), flushing, dizziness, reflex tachycardia or bradycardia, hypokalemia, ↑ intraocular pressure, local phlebitis. Contraindications: patients with glaucoma or ↑ intraocular pressure.
Labetalol Most hypertensive emergencies, especially aortic dissection and pheochromocytoma crisis.	Sympathetic blocker. Blocks alpha and beta-receptors. ↓ afterload; ↓ cardiac output; no effect on preload.	20–80 mg IV bolus over 2 min every 10 min (total dose 300 mg) or 0.5–2 mg/min IV infusion. Onset of action: 5–10 min. Duration: 2–6 h.	Side effects: bradycardia, heart block, worsened or new-onset HF. Contraindications: symptomatic bradycardia or heart block; acute HF; reactive airway disease; cocaine toxicity.

(continued on next page)

Table 3
(continued)

Medication/Indication	Action	Dosing Information	Nursing Implications (in Addition to Monitoring for Hypotension)
Esmolol Aortic dissection, perioperative HTN crises. Not for catecholamine excess.	Sympathetic blocker. Ultrarapid, short-acting beta-1 (cardioselective) blocker. ↓ cardiac output; no effect on preload or afterload.	80-mg bolus over 30 s, then 150 µg/kg/min IV infusion. Onset of action: 1–2 min. Duration: 10–20 min.	Requires intra-arterial BP monitoring. Side effects: bradycardia, heart block, worsened or new-onset HF; may cause thrombophlebitis and extravasation (including local necrosis). Contraindications: symptomatic bradycardia or heart block; acute HF; reactive airway disease; cocaine toxicity.
Phentolamine Catecholamine excess.	Sympathetic blocker. Nonselective alpha blocker. ↓ afterload; ↑ cardiac output. No effect on preload.	5–15-mg IV bolus. Onset of action: 1–2 min. Duration: 10–15 min.	Side effects: flushing, headache, reflex tachycardia.
Nicardipine Most hypertensive emergencies, including perioperative and postoperative HTN.	Calcium channel blocker, 3rd generation, dihydropyridine. Arterial vasodilator. No negative inotropic effects. ↓ afterload; ↑ cardiac output; no effect on preload.	Dose: 2–15 mg/h as IV infusion. Onset: 1–5 min. Duration: 15–120 min. Dose independent of body weight. Monitor and titrate to lowest dose.	Side effects: reflex tachycardia. Cautious use: patients with CHD (tachycardia can ↑ ischemia) or those with suspected GI bleeding.
Clevidipine Most hypertensive emergencies.	Calcium channel blocker. Relaxes smooth muscles; ↓ peripheral resistance. ↓ afterload; ↑ cardiac output; no effect on preload.	1–2 mg/h doubling the dose at 90-s intervals initially; later at 5–10-min intervals based on BP effect. Titrate to maximum 16 mg/h IV infusion. (Usual dose 4–6 mg/h). Onset of action: 1–4 min. Duration: 5–15 min.	May administer in a central or peripheral IV line. Side effects: Nausea, vomiting, headache, AF. Contraindications: persons with AF; those who have soy allergy.
Enalaprilat For HTN emergencies, especially acute HF.	ACE inhibitor. ↓ afterload; ↑ cardiac output; no effect on preload.	1.25–5 mg (over 2–5 min) every 6 h IV bolus. Onset of action: 15–30 min. Duration: 12–24 h.	Side effects: headache, nausea, cough, hyperkalemia, worsened kidney function. Contraindication: History of ACE-inhibitor allergy or angioedema.

Abbreviations: ACE, angiotensin-converting enzyme; AF, atrial fibrillation; BP, blood pressure; BUN, blood urea nitrogen; CABG, coronary artery bypass graft; CHD, coronary heart disease; GI, gastrointestinal; HF, heart failure; HTN, hypertension; ICP, intracranial pressure; IV, intravenous; ↑, increase; ↓, decrease; ↓↓, more of a decrease.
Data from Refs.[7,10,11]

Heart Failure

Burden of the condition

As with HTN, the prevalence of HF increases with age; about half of the adults with HF in the US are at least age 75.[12,13] It is generally considered a condition of elders.[14] HF is the leading cause of hospitalization for those age 65 and older.[6,14,15] At baseline, elders with HF are more likely to be women, to have preserved systolic function (ie, normal EF), and to have isolated systolic HTN as the precipitating cause of HF.[12] Younger adults with HF are more likely to be men, have systolic dysfunction, and to have an ischemic etiology.[12] However, of those elders who are admitted with HF, the percentage with systolic dysfunction is higher than among those in the community.[12,13]

Systolic HTN is the greatest risk factor for the development of HF, especially among women.[12,13] In addition to increased age and systolic HTN, risk factors for HF in the elderly include having coronary heart disease (CHD), AF, a widened pulse pressure, diabetes, chronic lung disease, kidney dysfunction, left ventricular hypertrophy (LVH), and obesity. Age-related changes to the CV system (eg, increased arterial and ventricular stiffness, impaired beta-adrenergic responsiveness), combined with age-related changes to the kidneys and lungs, place elders at risk for the development of HF.[12,13] These combined age-related effects and comorbid conditions also influence the ability of elders to compensate during an exacerbation of HF and their response to treatment during exacerbations.

Acute decompensation of HF

Acute decompensated heart failure (ADHF) is a clinical classification of rapidly worsening HF and is primarily diagnosed by a patient's signs and symptoms.[15,16] Approximately 80% of individuals with ADHF have chronic HF that acutely decompensates, known as "acute on chronic HF."[16,17] These patients typically present with a history of progressive, worsening chronic HF, usually with evidence of either systemic or pulmonary congestion.[15,16] The remaining 20% of patients with ADHF have new-onset HF.[16] During acute episodes, the renin-angiotensin-aldosterone system (RAAS) is activated, causing an increase in sodium and water retention by the kidneys, an increase in circulating blood volume, and an increase in venous pressure.[12,15] Fluid accumulates in the lung's interstitial and alveolar spaces, resulting in acutely elevated cardiac filling pressures.[15,16] These high-risk patients require immediate medical attention, are usually hospitalized in the ICU, and receive acute pharmacologic therapy.

Precipitating factors for ADHF

Decompensation is typically caused by one or more precipitants; rarely does ADHF occur because of a sudden decline in the structure or function of the heart.[15,16] Instead, decompensation is usually associated with worsening comorbid conditions (eg, worsening kidney function), a gradual decline in myocardial function, and/or persistent neurohormonal activation caused by the chronic underlying cardiac condition.[15,16] Reasons for decompensation may differ based on the type of HF a patient has. For example, the primary reason for decompensation in patients with reduced EF is impaired contractility (increased end-systolic volume), often due to ischemia.[12,13] Elderly patients who have increased systemic vascular resistance, higher norepinephrine levels, and impaired kidney function are more likely to go into acute HF, especially during times of ischemia.[12]

In contrast, the primary reason for decompensation in patients with preserved EF is inability to increase left ventricular (LV) stroke volume due to the presence of increased vascular stiffness, despite increased LV filling pressures.[12] This group experiences impaired relaxation of the LV, and thus has difficulty receiving blood into the ventricle. In the past, it was thought that transient systolic dysfunction, acute ischemia, or mitral regurgitation played the primary role in acute pulmonary edema in these patients. However, a more current view of the pathogenesis of acute pulmonary edema is that it is a consequence of markedly elevated SBP.[12,18] There are several pathophysiological mechanisms for decompensation in patients with preserved EF (abnormalities in ventricular diastole, vascular stiffness, circulatory volume overload, and atrial dysfunction) all more likely with advanced age.[12,18] Increases in LV mass and LV volume from long-standing HTN, diabetes, or obesity further compromise the patient.[12] Also, because LV relaxation is sensitive to changes in afterload and HR, patients can more easily decompensate during episodes of HTN or tachycardia.[12] **Box 1** provides a list of possible precipitants of ADHF.

Signs and symptoms of ADHF
Assessing symptoms of HF is challenging in elderly patients because they are more likely to attribute their symptoms to getting older, being deconditioned, or being obese. They are also unlikely to report exertional symptoms if they lead a sedentary life.[12] As with many CV conditions, their symptoms are also more likely to be atypical (eg, somnolence or malaise, weakness or confusion, irritability, anorexia, general abdominal complaints, sleep disturbance, or decreased activity).[12] However, nurses should be knowledgeable about the classic presentations of ADHF.

The *most common* presentation of ADHF includes pulmonary and systemic congestion *without* a decline in cardiac output.[15] In fact, many patients (30%–50%) who are evaluated in the emergency department or hospitalized for ADHF have systemic HTN (SBP>140 mm Hg) at the time of evaluation, not hypotension.[15] Cardinal signs and symptoms of ADHF include shortness of breath, congestion, and fatigue.[12,14,15] Congestion may occur as pulmonary congestion or as systemic congestion. Thus, nurses should keep in mind that pulmonary congestion *may* be present, even in the

---

Box 1
Precipitants for acute decompensated heart failure

- Ischemia (ACS)
- Worsening or uncontrolled HTN
- Dysrhythmias (eg, AF or atrial flutter)
- Valvular abnormalities (eg, mitral regurgitation)
- Comorbid conditions (eg, diabetes, thyroid disease, pulmonary disease, or new/worsening kidney disease)
- Infections (eg, chest infections, pneumonia, myocarditis, pericarditis, or endocarditis)
- Hematologic disorders (eg, severe anemia or bone marrow suppression)
- Nonadherence with medications or sodium/fluid restrictions (may be due to financial or knowledge factors)
- Cardiotoxic agents (alcohol or illicit drug use)
- Iatrogenic factors (agents that cause sodium or water retention; medications that are negative inotropes; sympathomimetic use [eg, pseudoepinephrine, ephedra, or amphetamines])

Abbreviations: ACS, acute coronary syndrome; AF, atrial fibrillation; HTN, hypertension.
Data from Refs.[12,15,16]

absence of rales/crackles or evidence of fluid on the chest radiograph.[14,15] Although not the majority, some patients present with low output (inadequate tissue perfusion). Symptoms of inadequate perfusion may be *more subtle* than those of congestion, especially in elders.[12] Therefore, nurses should be able to recognize the signs and symptoms of low output *promptly*, because cardiogenic shock may be imminent in patients who have low cardiac output.[12] **Table 4** lists the signs/symptoms of ADHF.

Diagnosis of ADHF

The diagnosis of ADHF is primarily based on the patient's clinical signs and symptoms.[14,15] However, there are some tests that are useful in confirming the diagnosis, assessing the severity of disease, and evaluating the results of therapy. Two sub-types of natriuretic peptides, B-type natriuretic peptide (BNP) and N-terminal pro-B-type natriuretic peptide (NT-proBNP), may be ordered to increase certainty about the diagnosis.[14,15] These naturally occurring hormones, secreted from the atria and ventricles

Table 4		
Signs and symptoms of acute decompensated heart failure		
Body Symptom	**Sign/Symptoms of Pulmonary and Systemic Congestion**	**Sign/Symptoms of Low Output (Inadequate Tissue Perfusion)**
General	Weight gain (or stable weight if anorexia present at baseline); excessive thirst or dry mouth; may be apprehensive.	Fatigue at rest, decreased exercise tolerance, weight loss, cachexia, temporary wasting, lethargy, and somnolence.
Cardiovascular	JVD, S_3 gallop, new-onset or increased mitral regurgitation, right ventricular heave, increased central venous pressure or right atrial pressure.	Absent JVD, decreased systolic BP (<85 mm Hg or if symptomatic), orthostatic BP and HR on standing, resting tachycardia, decreased mean arterial pressure, narrow pulse pressure, increased systemic vascular resistance, decreased temperature.
Pulmonary	Dyspnea on exertion, orthopnea, paroxysmal nocturnal dyspnea, nocturnal cough, rales, wheezes, pleural effusion, tachypnea, decreased oxygen saturations, pulmonary edema on chest x-ray.	Dyspnea *without* orthopnea or paroxysmal nocturnal dyspnea, dyspnea on exertion with *clear* breath sounds, *clear* chest x-ray, decreased oxygen consumption, decreased arterial oxygen saturation.
Gastrointestinal	Hepatomegaly, ascites, right upper quadrant tenderness, nausea, vomiting, diarrhea, anorexia, elevated liver function tests.	Early satiety, anorexia, increased liver function tests *without* hepatomegaly, right upper quadrant tenderness, nausea, vomiting, bright red blood per rectum.
Renal	Urine output may be increased if oral intake is increased; increased nocturia.	Increased blood BUN, increased Cr, oliguria or anuria; decreased serum sodium.
Extremities	Warm pitting peripheral edema, strong peripheral pulses.	Cool; absent, or nonpitting edema; weak peripheral pulses.

Abbreviations: BP, blood pressure; BUN, blood urea nitrogen; Cr, creatinine; JVD, jugular vein distension.
Data from Refs.[12,14–16]

as a result of cardiac dilation, have been found to be highly predictive in diagnosing patients with HF, regardless of whether they have a normal EF or low EF.[14,15] Both types of hormones increase with age, particularly in women, in obese individuals, and in those with kidney impairment.[15] Assay specificity is lower for elders, especially older women with preserved LV function (age 70–105 years), than for younger patients (18–69 years) with HF.[15] NT-proBNP has a longer half-life and in general runs about 4 times higher than BNP.[15] Despite these limitations in specificity, there are cut points for diagnosis. A BNP level greater than 500 pg/mL is considered diagnostic of ADHF.[15] The cut point for a positive diagnosis of ADHF by NT-proBNP testing is based on age: higher than 450 pg/mL for patients younger than 50, higher than 900 pg/mL for those age 50 to 75 years, and higher than 1800 pg/mL for those older than 74.[15] Although natriuretic peptides may be helpful in improving diagnostic certainty, the usefulness of serial measurement of these tests to reduce hospitalization or mortality is not well established.[14] Furthermore, current recommendations for the treatment of HF advise that natriuretic peptides may be useful in the outpatient setting to optimize medical therapy.[14] However, more research is needed before recommending widespread use.

Echocardiography is considered the gold standard noninvasive test for diagnosing and monitoring HF.[12,14,15] An echocardiogram provides information about both cardiac structure and function, including estimates of LVEF, wall motion abnormalities, and the integrity of the heart valves, all of which are helpful in sorting out the etiology of the HF. However, standard echocardiography is unable to distinguish diastolic dysfunction related to "normal" aging from HF.[12,14,15] Thus, it is best to combine standard echocardiography with Doppler imaging to ensure accurate assessment diastolic function.

Other diagnostic tests typically done for patients admitted with ADHF include chest radiograph (to rule out cardiac enlargement, pulmonary congestion, pleural effusion, pneumothorax, and/or the placement of cardiac devices), 12-lead ECG (to assess heart rate and rhythm or the presence of LVH or acute ischemia), and standard laboratory studies (serum electrolytes, including calcium, magnesium, and phosphorus, complete blood count, serum albumin, uric acid, liver function tests, and thyroid function studies).[14,15]

Treatment of ADHF

Primary treatment goals for patients admitted with ADHF include improving symptoms (especially symptoms of congestion and low output), restoring oxygenation, and optimizing volume status.[12,14,15] In addition, hospitalization provides an opportunity for the medical team to reevaluate the ongoing treatment regimen to ensure that the patient is receiving guideline-directed medical therapy for optimal short-term and long-term outcomes. **Box 2** lists the treatment goals for patients hospitalized with ADHF.

Many clinicians use a classification system to assign a clinical profile to patients with ADHF to guide pharmacologic therapy with IV diuretics, inotropes, and/or vasodilators. Classification systems differentiate clinical profiles based on the adequacy of tissue perfusion ("warm" vs "cold") and the degree of congestion ("wet" vs "dry").[14–16] The most frequent presentation of ADHF is the "warm and wet" clinical profile.[15,16] Patients with this profile should generally be treated with IV loop diuretics or an increased dose or increased frequency of oral diuretics, because of their congestion.[14–16] In addition to diuretics, vasodilators (such as nitroglycerin, sodium nitroprusside, or nesiritide) may be used for patients with this profile, as their BP generally permits use.[14–16] Patients with a second type of clinical profile, those who are "cold and wet," are also treated with IV loop diuretics because the etiology of hypoperfusion

---

Box 2
Treatment goals for acute decompensated heart failure

- Improve symptoms, especially those related to congestion and low output
- Restore oxygenation
- Optimize volume status
- Identify the etiology of the HF
- Identify and correct precipitating factors
- Optimize chronic therapy
- Minimize side effects of treatment regimen
- Identify which patients may benefit from revascularization and/or device therapy
- Identify which patients are candidates for anticoagulation therapy (high risk for thromboembolism)
- Educate patients and families concerning treatment regimen and self-assessment of HF
- Refer to a disease management program if available

Abbreviation: HF, heart failure.
Data from Refs.[12,14–16]

---

is likely to be congestion. However, diuretics may be minimally effective if perfusion to the kidneys is affected by the low output.[14–16] Regardless of the presence or absence of congestion, inotropes (eg, dopamine, dobutamine, or milrinone) are used for all patients classified as "cold" to assist with circulation.[14–16,19] The third profile, "warm and dry," is actually the "target" profile that is desired after treatment. However, if patients who present with ADHF have adequate perfusion and are without congestion, treatment should focus on searching for other causes of their HF (such as ACS, pulmonary embolus, infection, anemia, hypothyroidism, or depression).[14–16] In this case, they should not receive IV diuretics (to avoid hypotension). The final profile for hospitalized patients with ADHF is the "cold and dry" clinical profile, which is least prevalent. Inotropes are the treatment of choice because of the hypoperfusion ("the coldness").[14–16,19] Diuretics and vasodilators are not given because of the potential for marked hypotension or irreversible organ damage.[14–16] **Table 5** provides a summary of the clinical profiles and general treatment recommendations.

Regardless of which clinical profile the patient has, there are general principles that nurses should consider when administering IV diuretics, vasodilators, and inotropes to patients with ADHF. Generally considered first-line agents, IV loop diuretics should be given to all patients with evidence of fluid overload.[12,14–16] Administration by the IV route is preferred over the oral route because of better effectiveness and a faster clinical response (as rapidly as 15 minutes in some patients) with IV diuresis.[14–16,19] Symptomatic relief is generally obtained within 1 to 2 hours, compared with oral maintenance doses, which may take weeks to rid excess fluid.[15] If the patient has a history of chronic HF and decompensates acutely, the initial dose of IV diuretic should equal to or exceed their long-term oral daily dose.[14,16] Higher doses may be needed for those with kidney disease or those with severe fluid overload to gain symptomatic relief.[14,15] Current treatment guidelines for ADHF do not specify a preference for intermittent bolus injections of IV diuresis versus a continuous infusion.[14,15] Advantages of intermittent bolus injections include the convenience of administering the medication at a specific time and that continuous IV access is not required.[16,20] However,

Table 5
Classification clinical profiles and treatment of acute decompensated heart failure

Profile	Characteristics	Treatment
Cold and wet	Inadequate tissue perfusion	IV loop diuretic (not as effective if kidney perfusion is compromised)
	Congested	Inotropes (dopamine, dobutamine, or milrinone)
Warm and wet	Adequate tissue perfusion	IV loop diuretic
	Congested	Vasodilators (nitroglycerin, sodium nitroprusside, or nesiritide)
Cold and dry: least common profile	Inadequate tissue perfusion	Inotropes (as above)
	Not congested	Avoid use of diuretics and vasodilators due to profound hypotension or irreversible organ damage
Warm and dry: the target profile *after* treatment	Adequate tissue perfusion	Search for other causes of HF.
	Not congested	Avoid IV diuretics to prevent hypotension

Abbreviations: HF, heart failure; IV, intravenous.
Data from Refs.[12,14–16]

some patients do not respond to intermittent bolus injections; thus, a continuous infusion of a loop diuretic should be considered.[14–16,20] Advantages to a continuous infusion include a more constant delivery of the agent to the kidneys and less chance of causing prerenal azotemia, less chance of causing side effects from fluctuations in drug levels, and less chance of developing rebound sodium reabsorption if the drug were to drop below the therapeutic range.[16,20] Other recommendations for patients who do not respond to the initial dose of IV diuresis include increasing the dose of the loop diuretic, adding a second type of diuretic (thiazide) to work synergistically with the loop diuretic, implementing a sodium and fluid restriction for the patient, and consideration of ultrafiltration, if available at the facility.[14–16,20] In contrast, for patients who develop worsened kidney function after receiving IV diuresis, treatment options include a temporary dose decrease or discontinuation of the diuretic, use of vasodilator or inotrope therapy, or short-term hemodialysis may be considered for patients who have continued fluid volume overload in the setting of worsened kidney function.[16] **Table 6** gives information on IV diuretics used to treat ADHF.

Vasodilators, generally considered second-line agents, are best used for patients who have volume overload, yet normal or elevated BP (ideally an SBP of >110 mm Hg).[14–16,19] All IV vasodilators need to be administered by an infusion pump, and some facilities require invasive hemodynamic monitoring when administering some of these agents (such as sodium nitroprusside).[14–16] Inotropes are typically considered a third-line agent in some patients with ADHF because current guidelines deemphasize the use of inotropes as compared with vasodilators. However, IV inotropes are a good option for patients who have symptomatic hypotension (SBP<90 mm Hg) or borderline SBP who are unable to receive vasodilators safely. Inotropes help patients with severe systolic dysfunction, hypotension, or evidence of low cardiac output, with or without congestion, to maintain systemic perfusion and preserve end-organ performance.[14–16,19] **Table 6** also provides information on IV vasodilators and IV inotropes used to treat ADHF.

Table 6
Intravenous medications used to treat acute decompensated heart failure

Medication Class/Action(s)	Examples/Dose Recommendations	Side Effects	Nursing Implications
Loop diuretics ↑ urinary excretion of sodium, chloride, and water. ↓ circulating intravascular volume (↓ preload and central venous pressure). ↓ signs of fluid retention.	**Furosemide** Loading IV dose: 40 mg. Continuous IV infusion should be adjusted to CrCl; typically 10–40 mg/h. IV doses exceeding 300 mg/d in patients with ADHF have increased mortality. **Bumetanide** Loading IV dose: 1 mg. Maximum IV dose: 10 mg/d. Continuous IV infusion should be adjusted to CrCl; typically 0.5–2 mg/h. **Torsemide** Loading IV dose: 20 mg. Continuous IV infusion: typically 5–20 mg/h.	Most serious: If given too rapidly may cause symptomatic hypotension, worsened kidney function, serious serum electrolyte abnormalities. Most common: Worsened kidney function (↑ serum BUN, creatinine). Fluid volume deficit (hypovolemia, dehydration, orthostatic hypotension, dizziness, presyncope, syncope). Electrolyte imbalances (↓ potassium, sodium, calcium; metabolic alkalosis; ↑ glucose, lipid levels, uric acid). Less common: ototoxicity.	Monitor BP, HR, and cardiac rhythm every 1–2 h. Monitor signs and symptoms of congestion and changes in body weight. Daily weights, comparing to patient's dry weight (weight before decompensation). Monitor intake and output records. Monitor serum electrolytes. Report abnormal values to the medical team caring for the patient. Instruct patient to change positions slowly to avoid syncope. Monitor for ringing in the ears or hearing loss.

(continued on next page)

Table 6
(continued)

Medication Class/Action(s)	Examples/Dose Recommendations	Side Effects	Nursing Implications
Vasodilators ↓ BP (↓ preload and afterload by venous and arterial vasodilation). ↓ PCWP and CVP (by ↓ preload). ↓ SVR (afterload). All need to be administered by an IV infusion pump. Patients with a peripheral IV are at risk for infiltration and necrosis. Monitor BP, HR, and cardiac rhythm every 1–2 h. Need to wean vasodilators slowly to avoid rebound vasoconstriction.	**Nitroglycerin** Initial dose: 10–20 µg/min. Typical dose range: 5–200 µg/min. Adjustment increment: 10–20 µg/min every 5–15 min. Maximum dose: titrate up to a max of 200 µg/min. **Sodium nitroprusside** Initial dose: 0.2–0.3 µg/kg/min. Typical dose range: 0.5–5 µg/kg/min (usually 5–300 µg/min). Adjustment increment: 0.25–0.50 µg/kg/min every 5–15 min (while maintaining an SBP of >90 mm Hg or MAP >65 mm Hg). Maximum dose: 5 µg/kg/min. **Nesiritide** Initial loading (bolus) dose: 2 µg/kg. (May omit loading dose if there is concern for hypotension.) Followed by infusion of: 0.1 µg/kg/min. Adjustment increment: 0.005 µg/kg/min; bolus 1 µg/kg/min every 3 h to maximum dose. Maximum dose: 0.03 µg/kg/min.	Symptomatic hypotension (esp. if given with IV diuretic), headache, abdominal discomfort, reflex tachycardia, paradoxic bradycardia. May cause profound hypotension. Serious side effects: cyanide and thiocyanate toxicities especially in patients with liver or kidney impairment. Symptomatic hypotension (especially if given with IV diuretic), headache, worsening kidney function (dose dependent). Serious side effect: May worsen ischemia in patients with ACS.	May develop tolerance (decreased response to drug) if receiving a continuous infusion >24 h. Need to monitor patients for cyanide toxicity (change in mental status, muscle spasms, convulsions, hemodynamic instability, unexplained metabolic or lactic acidosis). Risk of toxicity ↓ if given at lower doses and used for <72 h. Should not be given to patients with acute cardiac ischemia (patients with ACS).

Inotropes

Dopamine

Sympathomimetic (↑ HR and CO). Effects are dose dependent. Best choice for "cold and dry" or those in cardiogenic shock.	Starting dose: 2 µg/kg/min (no loading dose). Adjustment increment: 0.005 µg/kg/min; bolus 1 µg/kg every 3 h to maximum dose of 10 µg/kg/min. Note: Low dose (<3 µg/kg/min) = ↑ urine output and sodium excretion. Moderate dose (3–5 µg/kg/min) = inotrope effect (↑ CO and SBP). High dose (>5 µg/kg/min) = vasopressor effect (↑ CO, BP; ↓ blood to kidneys and periphery).	Common side effect: Tachycardia, headache, nausea, ↓ urine output (with high doses). Serious side effect: tissue necrosis.	All should be given via an infusion pump. All should be started and stopped gradually (weaned). Frequent monitoring of BP, HR, and cardiac rhythm. Notify medical team if patient develops symptomatic hypotension or serious arrhythmia. Most (not all) complications are related to higher doses and/or longer lengths of time on IV inotropes.

(continued on next page)

Table 6
(continued)

Medication Class/Action(s)	Examples/Dose Recommendations	Side Effects	Nursing Implications
Dobutamine			
Synthetic catecholamine. Stimulates β_1 and β_2 adrenergic receptors (↑ HR, BP, and contractility). Dose dependent ↑ CO and ↓ PCWP.	Starting dose: 2–5 µg/kg/min (*no loading dose). Typical dose range: 2.5–20 µg/kg/min (side effects are dose dependent). Adjustment increment: 2.5–5 µg/kg/min every 5–15 min.	Common side effect: ↑ or ↓ BP, headache, tachycardia (more likely with this inotrope), nausea, fever. Serious side effect: hypersensitivity, increased myocardial ischemia, AF.	Best choice for patients who are "cold and dry" (SBP <90 mm Hg). Avoid in patients with ACS (due to ↑ HR and myocardial oxygen demand).
Milrinone			
Phodiesterase type-3 inhibitor. ↑ intracellular calcium concentration, myocardial contractility and myocardial relaxation. (↑ arterial and venous vasodilation, ↓ SVR and PVR, ↑ CO).	Initial loading dose: 50 µg/kg (may omit if a concern for hypotension). Starting infusion: 0.25 µg/kg/min. Typical dose range: 0.25–0.75 µg/kg/min. Adjustment increment: titration based on hemodynamic response (↑ CO and ↓ PCWP).	Common side effects: Tachycardia, hypotension (more likely with this inotrope), atrial and ventricular arrhythmias. Serious side effects: Long-term use associated with decreased survival (cardiac arrest).	Best choice for patients who are "cold and wet" (SBP <90 mm Hg). Better choice for patients who are on beta-blockers (compared to dobutamine which stimulates beta-receptors).

Abbreviations: ACS, acute coronary syndrome; AF, atrial fibrillation; BP, blood pressure; CO, cardiac output; CrCl, creatinine clearance; CVP, central venous pressure; HR, heart rate; IV, intravenous; PCWP, pulmonary capillary wedge pressure; PVR, peripheral vascular resistance; SBP, systolic blood pressure; SVR, systemic vascular resistance; ↑, increase; ↓, decrease.
Data from Refs.[12,14–16,19]

Other miscellaneous medications for ADHF

Traditionally, IV morphine has been used to stabilize patients with acute pulmonary edema. However, recent studies have shown that morphine given to acutely ill patients with ADHF is associated with worse outcomes (longer hospital stay, need for mechanical ventilation, need for ICU, and higher overall mortality).[15] The mechanism related to this association is unclear. Thus, the current guidelines for treatment of ADHF indicate that morphine should be used cautiously, especially in those with impaired respiratory drive or altered mental status.[15,16] If used at all, morphine should be given at low doses (2.5–5.0 mg) and the patient should be monitored for side effects (eg, hypotension, bradycardia, advanced heart block, and carbon dioxide retention).[15]

Digoxin is generally not used in the acute setting of ADHF. However, some patients may be on digoxin before hospitalization (eg, those with preexisting HF or AF) and may continue to receive the medication throughout their hospital stay. Although digoxin helps decrease symptoms of HF, the use of this agent has not been shown to improve survival, especially in the acute setting. The use of digoxin in managing patients with ADHF is not addressed in the current treatment guidelines.[15,16] If digoxin is used, doses are generally lower than previously advised, especially in elders or those with kidney dysfunction.[12] This is largely due to an analysis of the Digitalis Investigation Group (DIG) study, which showed that the maximum benefit of digoxin was evident at serum levels of 0.5 to 0.8 ng/mL.[12,21] In fact, digoxin levels greater than 1.2 (previously thought to be "therapeutic") were associated with increased mortality.[12,21] Thus, a dosage of 0.125 mg daily is adequate for most elders with normal kidney function; and a lower dosage (0.125 mg 1–3 times per week) is appropriate for those with impaired kidney function.[12,22]

Aspirin is also not indicated for ADHF, unless the patient has a known history of CHD or is experiencing acute cardiac ischemia. If aspirin is given, the lowest dosage (81 mg daily) should be used to minimize the chance of bleeding or interaction with angiotensin-converting enzyme (ACE) inhibitors.[15,16]

Maintenance therapies in the setting of ADHF

Medications given in the acute ICU setting for ADHF are generally given to improve the patient's symptoms and hemodynamics. However, hospitalization also offers an opportunity to optimize long-term therapy for patients transitioning from the hospital to the community. Long-term benefits of maintenance therapies include attenuating (slowing down) the disease process, decreasing the chances of rehospitalization, and improving survival. Maintenance therapy includes ACE inhibitors (or angiotensin receptor blockers [ARBs], if allergic), beta-adrenergic antagonists (beta-blockers), loop diuretics, aldosterone antagonists, and digoxin (for some patients with reduced LVEF).[12,14,15] However, nurses should be aware that elders are at increased risk for side effects from these therapies. For example, because elders have a greater likelihood of underlying chronic kidney disease and renal artery stenosis, they are at an increased risk of orthostatic hypotension or worsened kidney function when given ACE inhibitors, especially if patients take nonsteroidal anti-inflammatory drugs.[12] Elders are also at higher risk for kidney dysfunction and electrolyte abnormalities with the use of diuretic therapy.[12,14] Thus, the lowest possible dose of diuretic should be used, while still maintaining euvolemia (normal fluid volume status).[12] Thus, the inpatient setting may provide an opportunity for close monitoring that would otherwise not be available as an outpatient to monitor for these potential side effects (especially if patients have borderline or low BP, a low HR, or have borderline electrolyte abnormalities). **Box 3** provides pearls for starting or up-titrating maintenance therapies for patients who have been hospitalized for ADHF.

Box 3
Pearls for starting or up titrating maintenance therapies

- ACE-inhibitors (or ARBs) can be started (or up-titrated) if the kidney function is stable.
- Doses of ACE inhibitors (or ARBs) can be adjusted more frequently in the in-hospital setting, because side effects and laboratory findings can be monitored more closely.
- Generally, patients should be on target doses of ACE inhibitors (or ARBs) and on a low-dose diuretic before starting beta-blocker therapy for chronic HF.
- For patients who are newly diagnosed with HF, beta-blocker therapy should be started at the lowest dose 24 hours before hospital discharge, after the volume status is optimized, successful conversion of IV to oral diuretics has occurred, and after all vasodilators or inotropes have been weaned off.
- Patients on chronic beta-blocker therapy who are not yet at target doses may have their beta-blocker up-titrated 24 hours before hospital discharge (with the same conditions as above).
- After hospital discharge uptitration of beta-blocker and ACE-inhibitor therapy should occur every 2 to 4 weeks during a face-to-face visit to allow for assessment of vital signs and fluid volume.

Abbreviations: ACE, angiotensin-converting enzyme; ARB, angiotensin receptor blocker; HF, heart failure; IV, intravenous.
Data from Lindenfeld J, Albert NM, Boehmer JP. Heart Failure Society of America, executive summary: HFSA 2010 comprehensive heart failure practice guideline. J Card Fail 2010;16(6):e1–194; and Coons JC, McGraw M, Murali S. Pharmacotherapy for acute heart failure syndromes. Am J Health Syst Pharm 2011;68:21–35.

In rare circumstances, a patient's baseline therapy may have to be temporarily discontinued when they are admitted for ADHF. For example, if the patient with chronic HF is admitted with cardiogenic shock, refractory volume overload, or symptomatic bradycardia, then it would be appropriate to temporarily discontinue or give half their usual dose of beta-blocker (as opposed to complete discontinuation of the medication).[15] Also if the patient's SBP is lower than 80 mm Hg, is experiencing symptomatic hypotension, or has a markedly elevated creatinine compared with baseline, ACE inhibitor (or ARB) therapy should be reduced or temporarily discontinued until kidney function improves.[15] Finally, if a patient's kidney function dramatically worsens or their potassium become markedly elevated (>5.5 mEq/L) aldosterone antagonists (spironolactone or eplerenone) should be temporarily discontinued until the potassium has normalized or the kidney function has returned to baseline.[15]

Acute Coronary Syndrome (ACS)

Elders in the ICU are at an increased risk for acute cardiac ischemia, either from ACS or from the physiologic stress to the heart from other acute illnesses. Some patients with ACS have a history of stable angina that escalates prior to the event; others have no prior symptoms.

The diagnosis of ACS is an umbrella term that includes patients with unstable angina (UA), non–ST-Segment-Elevation MI (NSTEMI), or ST-Segment-Elevation MI (STEMI). UA refers to acute ischemic symptoms that increase in frequency and severity over time, often occurring at rest, either due to an increased demand for myocardial oxygen or a decreased supply (subtotal occlusion) of one or more coronary arteries.[6] The ischemia is transient and reversible, thus does not result in necrosis (death) of the myocardial tissue as with MI.[6] In contrast, an MI involves a total occlusion of at least one coronary artery, resulting in irreversible necrosis of the tissue that is supplied by the infarct-related artery. An STEMI is diagnosed if a symptomatic patient's 12-lead ECG has acute ST-segment elevation in 2 or more contiguous leads; whereas, patients who have ischemic symptoms without ST-segment elevation on their 12-lead ECG, yet rule in for an MI by cardiac enzymes (eg, creatine kinase MB [CK-MB] or troponin levels), are classified as NSTE MI.

Burden of the condition in elders

As individuals age, they are at greater risk for having an ACS event.[23,24] The median age for first-time MI in the United States is approximately 65 for men and 74 for women.[5] Furthermore, 35% of all MIs occur in persons 75 and older; 11% occurring in persons 85 and older.[23] Although the absolute numbers of patients with STEMI increases with age, elders are more likely to have an NSTE MI.[24] This is because elders are more likely to have complex calcified CHD, prior revascularization, and ACS due to other (secondary) conditions (eg, pneumonia, gastrointestinal bleeding, or sepsis).[23,24]

Advanced age is also an independent predictor for complications following an ACS event, including a higher risk of HF, bleeding, mechanical complications, and death.[24] In addition, ACS accounts for 35% of all deaths in adults 65 years and older, which increases sharply after the age of 75.[24] However, evidence-based treatment has been shown to improve mortality and morbidity in elderly patients with ACS, although not equal the outcomes of younger patients.[23,24] Possible reasons for worse outcomes in elders include longer delays in seeking care, a higher burden of underlying CHD (often undiagnosed), more end-organ damage, and more comorbid conditions, all of which influence the effectiveness of treatment options.[23]

Signs and symptoms of ACS

Chest pain is the most common symptom of ACS. However, as individuals age, they are more likely to have atypical symptoms, such as dyspnea, diaphoresis, nausea and vomiting, unusual fatigue, and syncope.[23] Thus, some elders may attribute atypical symptoms of ACS to other bodily conditions. Furthermore, elders are also more likely to have silent ischemia (no symptoms) with their ACS event compared with younger patients.[23] Symptoms of NSTEMI ACS usually manifest in 1 of 3 ways: (1) as rest angina (angina at rest, usually longer than 20 minutes), (2) new-onset angina (usually markedly limiting the person's activities), or (3) as progressively increasing angina (increased frequency, increased duration, or a lower threshold of what precipitates symptoms) in patients with preexisting CHD.[25]

Evaluation of ACS

Initial evaluation of patients with known or suspected ischemia should include a focused history (current symptoms, CV risk factors, and past medical history) and physical examination (check HR, BP, heart rhythm, heart and lung sounds, peripheral pulses, and presence of peripheral edema). In addition, all patients with known or suspected ischemia should have a 12-lead ECG performed within 10 minutes of hospital presentation. While obtaining a 12-lead ECG, the patient should be given aspirin (160–325 mg, nonenteric coated), unless contraindicated.[25] Aspirin should not be held while awaiting the 12-lead ECG. Unfortunately, many elderly patients, especially women or those with atypical symptoms, experience delay in receiving ECGs within the desired 10-minute time frame. In addition, elderly patients are more likely to have nondiagnostic ECGs or ECGs with abnormal baseline findings (eg, LVH, AF, bundle branch block, paced rhythms, or a prior MI), which confound the ability to detect acute ST-segment/T-wave changes.[23] If the first ECG is nondiagnostic, yet the patient remains highly symptomatic, additional ECGs may be done every 15 to

Table 7
Pharmacologic treatment for patients with ACS

Medication/ Use in ACS	Indication	Nursing Implications
NTG Anti-ischemic therapy.	Sublingual NTG 0.4 mg every 5 min up to 3 doses to treat ongoing ischemic discomfort. If symptoms continue after 3 sublingual NTGs, then assess the need for IV nitroglycerin. Intravenous NTG to treat persistent ischemia, pulmonary congestion, or HTN associated with the first 48 h of the ACS event.	Monitor for BP/HR for hypotension and tachycardia. Caution the patient that he or she may experience a headache. Treat headache with prn pain medications. Tolerance may develop in patients who have received >24 h of continuous IV NTG. For those who require IV NTG beyond 24 h, an increase of dose may be needed to maintain the anti-ischemic effect. Patients who have been symptom free for 12–24 h after IV NTG may be converted to oral or topical NTG. Contraindications: SBP <90 mm Hg or BP ≥30 mm Hg lower than their baseline, severe bradycardia (HR <50/min), tachycardia (HR>100/min) in the absence of symptomatic HF or RV infarct. Should not be given in patients who have received a phosphodiesterase inhibitor for erectile dysfunction within 24 h of sildenafil or 48 h of tadalafil use. The time frame for vardenafil has not been established.
Beta-blocker therapy Anti-ischemic, anti-arrhythmic, mortality reduction.	Oral beta-blocker therapy should be given within the first 24 h of an ACS event. IV beta-blockers may be considered for ongoing ischemic symptoms, especially with concurrent tachycardia or HTN. Nondihydropyridine calcium channel blockers (verapamil or diltiazem) may be given if beta-blockers are not tolerated or are contraindicated (except if severe LV dysfunction or other contraindications).	Monitor the patient's HR, BP, and heart rhythm. Lower doses may be needed initially for elders to evaluate the patient's response (due to the high first-pass effect in the liver and due to age-related changes to baroreceptors and beta-adrenergic receptors in the body). Contraindications: signs of HF, evidence of low output state (marked hypotension), symptomatic bradycardia, advanced heart block (2nd-degree or 3rd-degree AV block), active asthma or reactive airway disease.
ACE inhibitor therapy ↓ ventricular remodeling. ↑ long-term survival.	Oral ACE inhibitor within first 24 h if the patient has pulmonary congestion, LVEF ≤40%. Substitute: ARB.	Monitor the patient's HR, BP, and heart rhythm. Watch for hyperkalemia or a decline in kidney function in elders, especially those with underlying kidney impairment. Contraindications: SBP <100 mg Hg or BP ≥30 mm Hg below their baseline.

Antiplatelet therapy (aspirin, clopidogrel, prasugrel, or tigarelor).	Aspirin 160–325 mg, nonenteric coated should be chewed at the time of presentation and given orally daily thereafter (100–325 mg). Substitute: clopidogrel 75 mg daily (if aspirin allergy). Dual antiplatelet therapy (aspirin + clopidogrel, prasugrel, or tigarelor) should be considered for those having an early invasive approach (cardiac catheterization within 48 h).	Monitor patients for bleeding. When using dual antiplatelet therapy, aspirin doses should be $\leq$100 mg daily due to the increased risk of bleeding. Prasugrel is contraindicated in patients $\geq$75 y due to ↑ risk of death and intracranial bleeding.
Intravenous glycoprotein IIb/IIIa inhibitors	Eptifibatide: Weight-based bolus of 180 µg/kg and infusion of 2.0 µg/kg/min. Infusion should be adjusted if CrCl <50 mL/min to 1.0 µg/kg/min. Tirofiban: Weight-based bolus of 12 µg/kg and infusion of 0.1 µg/kg/min. Should be adjusted for kidney function (CrCl <30 mL/min) to bolus of 6 µg/kg and infusion of 0.05 µg/kg/min.	Calculate the patient's CrCl each day to verify that the patient is on the proper dose. Monitor the patient for bleeding. Increased bleeding is seen with elderly patients, especially if not properly weight adjusted or dose adjusted based on CrCl. Bleeding risk also increases with the number of antithrombin and antiplatelet agents given concurrently.
Antithrombin therapy (heparin)	Unfractionated heparin: weight-based bolus of 60 µg/kg and infusion of 12 µg/kg/min. Maximum bolus 4000 units and infusion of 900 u/h or 5000-unit bolus and infusion of 1000 u/h if patient weighs >100 kg. LMWH: weight-based dose of 1 mg/kg every 12 h. Adjustment in infusion for kidney function. If CrCl <30 mL/min, then 1 mg/kg subcutaneously every 24 h.	Monitor the patient for bleeding. Every elderly patient should have CrCl calculated every day. Patients are at ↑ risk for bleeding if altered kidney function. Alterations in body composition and protein levels in elders may result in overestimation of heparin dosing.

Abbreviations: ACE, angiotensin-converting enzyme; ACS, acute coronary syndrome; ARB, angiotensin receptor blocker; AV, atrioventricular; BP, blood pressure; CO, cardiac output; CrCl, creatinine clearance; CVP, central venous pressure; HR, heart rate; IV, intravenous; LMWH, low molecular weight heparin; LVEF, left ventricular ejection fraction; NTG, nitroglycerin; prn, as needed; RV, right ventricular; SBP, systolic blood pressure; u/h, units per hour; ↑, increase; ↓, decrease.

Data from Refs.[24–26]

30 minutes to detect possible ST-T-wave changes.[25] It is also important to obtain serial cardiac biomarkers (CK total, CK-MB, and troponin [the preferred biomarker]) to see if the patient has ruled in for an MI.[25] However, troponin levels could be elevated for reasons other than ACS (eg, myocardial contusion, sepsis, pulmonary embolus, stroke, or advanced kidney disease).[1,23]

Treatment of ACS

Studies have shown that many elders experiencing an ACS event do not receive evidence-based treatment.[23–25] As a result, in 2007 the American Heart Association (AHA) published a 2-part scientific statement on acute coronary care in the elderly, specifically addressing the care of elders suffering from NSTE ACS (Part I) and STEMI (Part II).[24,25] In addition, the latest AHA guidelines for ACS and STEMI also include a special groups section for treating older adults.[26,27]

All patients diagnosed with ACS who have continuing symptoms or hemodynamic instability should be admitted for at least 24 hours to the ICU.[25] These patients should receive continuous ECG monitoring for detection of arrhythmias, frequent assessments of vital signs and mental status, and continuous ST-segment monitoring (if available) to detect recurrent ischemia.[25] The most sensitive leads for viewing the infarct-related artery include Lead III for the right coronary artery, Lead V3 for the left anterior descending artery, and Lead V5 for the lateral and left circumflex artery. If the patient has ST-segment depression or elevation as the baseline, adjustments may be made to the ECG alarm settings to account for the baseline abnormalities. In addition, each patient should have access to defibrillation by the health care team if the patient experiences ventricular fibrillation.[25] If the patient does not have major complications within the first 24 hours, he or she may be moved out of the ICU. Examples of major complications include sustained ventricular arrhythmias, sinus tachycardia, high-grade atrioventricular block, sustained hypotension, recurrent ischemia (documented by symptoms or ST-segment deviation), new mitral regurgitation, or HF, any of which would keep the patient in the ICU.[25]

In addition, patients should receive supplemental oxygen by nasal cannula or facial mask if they have oxygen saturation less than 90%, are experiencing respiratory distress, or have other high-risk features for respiratory compromise.[25] Beyond continuous ECG monitoring and oxygen, treatment recommendations for elders with ACS are extrapolated from data with younger patients because most clinical trials have not included patients older than 75. In the ACS trials that have included elders, subgroup analysis has shown that in-hospital mortality decreases significantly as the number of recommended therapies given in the acute setting increases (eg, early use of aspirin, nitroglycerin, beta-blockers, ACE-inhibitors, heparin, glycoprotein IIb/IIIa inhibitors with percutaneous coronary intervention [PCI], and early cardiac catheterization [<48 hours]).[23] In fact, adults 75 and older with positive troponin levels (eg, NSTE MI) have been shown to gain a greater absolute benefit with an early invasive strategy (cardiac catheterization within 48 hours) compared with younger adults, mainly because of the much worse outcomes for elders who are treated more conservatively.[23] **Table 7** lists the recommended pharmacologic agents for treating patients with NSTE MI and UA.

Treatment of STEMI should include urgent reperfusion therapy.[23] Prompt reperfusion therapy (PCI within 90 minutes or fibrinolytic therapy within 30 minutes of hospital arrival) has shown a clear mortality benefit compared with not receiving reperfusion therapy, even for patients up to age 85.[23,25] Selection of reperfusion therapy generally favors PCI (vs fibrinolytic therapy).[23,25] However, the choice of reperfusion therapy also depends on risks and benefits for the individual patient, the time that symptoms began, and availability within the facility at the time of patient presentation.[23,25] PCI is especially beneficial in elders with cardiogenic shock, prior stroke, large anterior infarcts, or those who present later in their symptom course (>6 hours).[23] Benefits of urgent PCI include reduction in ischemic events and need for infarct-related artery revascularization, improved 30-day survival, and lower risk of hemorrhagic stroke at 30 days.[23]

Monitoring elders for bleeding
Several of the therapies (eg, antiplatelet and antithrombin agents) used to treat ACS have an accompanied risk of bleeding. With elders, bleeding is a function of age, comorbid conditions (eg, impaired kidney function, anemia as a baseline, diabetes, low body weight, prior history of bleeding, alterations in hemostatic factors that help individuals clot) and concomitant medication use.[23,27] Furthermore, bleeding is also related to excess dosing due to small body size and lower creatinine clearance.[24,27] Kidney function should be determined by calculating the patient's creatinine clearance, rather than using the serum creatinine. Nurses should also be diligent in monitoring elders for bleeding when these agents are given. Signs of bleeding may be more subtle and, if present, elders may downplay the symptoms. If a bleed is noted, the nurse should stop the offending agent (if known) and notify the medical team.

SUMMARY

Nurses working in the ICU will frequently encounter elderly patients with CV conditions, either as the primary or secondary diagnosis. However, it is challenging to distinguish between pathology of disease and physiologic changes due to aging. Nurses need to assess patients carefully because signs and symptoms are more likely to be more subtle or atypical in elders as compared with younger patients. Nurses also should monitor elderly patients more closely to watch for side effects of medications, especially if underlying kidney or liver impairment exists. Finally, although elders may be at increased risk for side effects of therapy, studies have shown that patients in their advanced years have the most benefit to gain with use of guideline-directed medical therapy.

REFERENCES

1. Pisani MA. Considerations in caring for the critically ill older patient. J Intensive Care Med 2009;24(2):83–95.
2. Suttner SW, Piper SN, Boldt J. The heart in the elderly critically ill patient. Curr Opin Crit Care 2002;8:389–94.
3. Marik PE. Management of the critically ill geriatric patient. Crit Care Med 2006; 34(9):S176–82.
4. Wright JD, Hughes JP, Ostchega Y, et al. Mean systolic and diastolic blood pressure in adults aged 18 and over in the United States, 2001-2008. Natl Health Stat Report 2011;35:1–22, 24.
5. Aronow WS, Fleg JL, Pepine CJ, et al. ACCF/AHA 2011 expert consensus document on hypertension in the elderly: a report of the American College of Cardiology Foundation Task Force on Clinical Expert Consensus Documents. J Am Coll Cardiol 2011;57:2037–114.
6. Go AS, Mozaffarian D, Roger VL, et al. Heart disease and stroke statistics—2013 update: a report from the American Heart Association. Circulation 2013;127: e6–245.

7. Johnson W, Nguyen ML, Patel R. Hypertension crisis in the emergency department. Cardiol Clin 2012;30:533–43.
8. Thomas L. Managing hypertensive emergencies in the emergency department. Can Fam Physician 2011;57:1137–41.
9. Lehman LH, Saeed M, Talmor D, et al. Methods of blood pressure measurement in the ICU. Crit Care Med 2013;41(1):34–40.
10. Slama M, Modeliar SS. Hypertension in the intensive care unit. Curr Opin Cardiol 2006;21:279–87.
11. Feldstein C. Management of hypertensive crises. Am J Ther 2007;14:135–9.
12. Maurer MS, Kitzman D. Essentials of cardiovascular care in older adults (ECCOA) curriculum. Heart Failure in older adults. Available at: http://www.cardiosource.org/ACC/ACC-Membership/Member-Sections-and-Councils/~/media/Files/ACC/Member%20Section%20Documents/ECCOA/Heart%20Failure%20in%20Older%20Adults%20%20Case%201%20of%203.ashx. Accessed September 29, 2013.
13. Kannel WB. Incidence and epidemiology of heart failure. Heart Fail Rev 2000;5:167–73.
14. Yancy CW, Jessup M, Bozkurt B, et al. 2013 ACCF/AHA guideline for the management of heart failure: a report of the American College of Cardiology Foundation/American Heart Association Task Force on practice guidelines. J Am Coll Cardiol 2013;62(16):1495–539.
15. Lindenfeld J, Albert NM, Boehmer JP. Heart Failure Society of America, executive summary: HFSA 2010 comprehensive heart failure practice guideline. J Card Fail 2010;16(6):e1–194.
16. Coons JC, McGraw M, Murali S. Pharmacotherapy for acute heart failure syndromes. Am J Health Syst Pharm 2011;68:21–35.
17. Gheorghiade M, Pang PS. Acute heart failure syndromes. J Am Coll Cardiol 2009;53:557–73.
18. Gandi SK, Powers JC, Nomeir AM, et al. The pathogenesis of acute pulmonary edema associated with hypertension. N Engl J Med 2001;344:17–22.
19. Coons JC, Seidl E. Cardiovascular pharmacotherapy update for the intensive care unit. Crit Care Nurs Q 2007;30(1):44–57.
20. Felker GM, Lee KL, Bull DA, et al. Diuretic strategies in patients with acute decompensated heart failure. N Engl J Med 2011;364:797–805.
21. Rich MW, McSherry F, Williford WO, et al. Effect of age on mortality, hospitalizations and response to digoxin in patients with heart failure: the DIG study. J Am Coll Cardiol 2001;38:806–13.
22. Rathore SS, Curtis JP, Wang Y, et al. Association of serum digoxin concentration and outcomes in patients with heart failure. J Am Med Assoc 2003;289:871–8.
23. Alexander K, Alpert J, Gharacholou M, et al. Essentials of cardiovascular care in older adults (ECCOA) curriculum. Overview: acute coronary syndromes in older adults. Available at: http://www.cardiosource.org/ACC/ACC-Membership/Member-Sections-and-Councils/~/media/Files/ACC/Member%20Section%20Documents/ECCOA/Acute%20Coronary%20Syndromes%20in%20Older%20Adults%20Overview.ashx. Accessed September 29, 2013.
24. Alexander KP, Newby LK, Cannon CP, et al. Acute coronary care in the elderly, Part 1: non-ST-Segment-Elevation acute coronary syndromes a scientific statement for healthcare professionals from the American Heart Association Council on Clinical Cardiology. Circulation 2007;115:2549–69.
25. Anderson JL, Adams CD, Antman EM, et al. 2012 ACCF/AHA focused update incorporated into the ACCF/AHA 2007 guidelines for the management of patients

with unstable angina/non-ST-elevation myocardial infarction: a report of the ACCF/AHA task force on practice guidelines. Circulation 2013;127:e663–828.

26. Alexander KP, Newby K, Armstrong PW, et al. Acute coronary care in the elderly, Part II: ST-segment-elevation myocardial infarction. A scientific statement for healthcare professionals from the American Heart Association Council on Clinical Cardiology. Circulation 2007;115:2570–89.

27. Alexander KP, Chen AY, Roe MT, et al. Excess dosing of anti-platelet and anti-thrombin agents in the treatment of non-ST segment elevation acute coronary syndromes. J Am Med Assoc 2005;294:3108–16.

Pulmonary Issues in the Older Adult

Delia E. Frederick, MSN, RN

KEYWORDS

- Older adults • Pulmonary issues • Effects of aging • Pneumonia
- Chronic obstructive pulmonary disease

KEY POINTS

- Overall body changes in muscular strength, skeletal structure, and mobility, in addition to cardiovascular function, result in changes in pulmonary function.
- Decreased thirst response, and less moisture within the mucous membranes of the upper and lower respiratory tract contribute to thickened mucus.
- Community-acquired pneumonia and chronic obstructive pulmonary disease are typical respiratory diseases in older adults.

INTRODUCTION

Pulmonary diseases are not the highest ranked reasons for admission to hospital, nor are they the principal reason for death in the United States. Pulmonary complications are of concern for all individuals admitted to an intensive care unit (ICU). Chronic lower respiratory diseases result in the deaths of only 6.2% of adults older than 65 years, and deaths attributable to influenza and pneumonia occur in of 2.6% of adults older than 65. Morbidity for chronic lower respiratory diseases is 6.4%.[1]

Nevertheless, older adults do have anatomic and physiologic changes that adversely affect the protective mechanisms for the pulmonary system.[2] Some of the changes nurses see in older adults are due to normal aging processes, but others are related to disease processes. It is imperative that nurses should not assume that alterations in pulmonary status are due to aging, and thus fail to intervene to correct the pulmonary issue. The purpose of this article is to review the changes that occur with aging and elucidate their effects on the pulmonary system. Interventions to deter complications and recognize respiratory distress are also provided.

The author has nothing to disclose.
School of Nursing, The University of North Carolina at Greensboro, Unit #9, 44 White Oak Street, Franklin, NC 28734, USA
E-mail address: defreder@uncg.edu

ANATOMY OF THE PULMONARY SYSTEM

The anatomy of the pulmonary system begins with the upper airway. The nose and mouth are entrances for air into the lungs. Atmospheric air is warmed and moistened as it courses through the nares. Adequate moisture of breathed air depends on a well-hydrated individual.[3]

The upper respiratory tract has 2 protective mechanisms to prevent foreign matter from entering the lower respiratory tract. The sneeze is a reflexive action that clears the upper airway when the presence of foreign matter enters the nose. This reflex is in place from the neonatal period until well into old age. The second protective mechanism is cilia within the posterior portion of the nares. Cilia are fine hairs that trap large foreign matter to prevent its entry into the lower respiratory tract. The cilia propel matter into the pharynx to be coughed out or swallowed. In a healthy older adult there is no decrease in the cough reflex.[3–5]

The pharynx has protective mechanisms in place to prevent aspiration of foreign matter into the lower respiratory tract. At the entrance to the lower respiratory tract, the tracheal opening, the glottis, is covered by the epiglottis during swallowing or at any time foreign matter makes contact with the glottis. This closure is a reflexive response that depends on cranial nerves IX (glossopharyngeal), X (vagus), and XII (hypoglossal). Effective swallowing is the result of coordination of these cranial nerves as well as many muscles, the cerebral cortex, the brainstem, and the cerebellum.[3,6]

The lower respiratory tract is enclosed in the thoracic cavity. The pulmonary system shares space with the heart and its structures. The skeletal structures of the thoracic cavity consist of an anterior sternum and a posterior vertebral column joined together by 12 pairs of curved ribs. Intercostal muscles allow for the movement of the skeletal structure necessary for inhalation and exhalation. In aging, reduced muscular strength or skeletal changes in the thorax can affect breathing even in the presence of healthy lung tissue.[2,4]

The trachea branches into 2 bronchi, then into the right and left lung fields. The right bronchus is straighter and more in line with the trachea, thus the risk of foreign-matter aspiration is more likely to occur in the right lung. The lungs are divided into lobes, of which there are 3 on the right and 2 on the left. The major lung fields are best auscultated on the back. It is important to assess lung sounds in all lung fields. Macrophages within the alveolar clusters consume foreign matter and bacteria that reach the terminal structures of the lungs. Gas exchange occurs at the alveolar-capillary membrane. The overall purpose of the pulmonary system is to deliver oxygen to the alveoli for diffusion into the bloodstream.[3,4]

ASSESSMENT OF THE PULMONARY SYSTEM

Respiratory rate provides a primary tool for determining homeostasis in individuals. The rate and effort of respirations in the older adult should be monitored, in addition to meticulous auscultation of lung sounds for abnormality. Tachypnea is an indication of hypercarbia, chemical irritation of the airways, or edema within the alveolar-capillary membrane tissue.[6] A full set of vital signs, including level of consciousness, is indicated to ensure stable oxygenation. Confusion, agitation, or both can indicate hypoxia. Tachycardia can be a sign of hypoxia.

Laboratory values are useful for evaluating pulmonary status.[7] Admission laboratory values may alert the nurse to potential risks of respiratory complications for an individual. Venous CO_2 can be referenced for metabolic processes in the absence of arterial blood gas. Fasting hyperglycemia on admission laboratory data has been found to be associated with higher rates of mortality in the presence of pneumonia.[8] An arterial blood gas indicates acid-base balance within the individual. Respiratory failure is indicated by a Pao_2 of less than 50 mm Hg and a $Paco_2$ of greater than 50 mm Hg. Brain natriuretic peptide (BNP) is a hormone secreted in response to elevated blood volume. Values of BNP higher than 100 μg/L indicate heart failure (**Table 1**).[6]

AGE-RELATED CHANGES THAT AFFECT THE PULMONARY SYSTEM

Older adults have a decreased thirst response, and thus may have less moisture within the mucous membranes of the upper and lower respiratory tracts. Poor hydration contributes to thickened mucus and increases the risk of the older adult being unable to clear sputum from the nose or lungs.[3] Older adults' intake and output, as well as blood urea nitrogen (BUN) and creatinine, indicate homeostasis of fluid volume. Excessive fluid volume impairs gas exchange at the alveolar-capillary interface.[6]

In older adults who have aspiration risk resulting from neurologic deficits, the cough response may be reduced. One small study of healthy older adults in a comparison with young healthy adults found a lower frequency of cough reflex in the older adults by a factor of one-third.[5] Speech volume and number of words spoken are affected by the volume of air within the lungs and the strength of the thoracic structures. The slow pace and length of idea delivery may suggest decreased cognition or may be attributed solely to the respiratory effort required to speak. Close attention to speech is needed to identify the effort of breathing in relation to decreased thinking in the older adult. Acute cognitive deficits may be related to hypoxia.[9]

Dysphagia in older adults can increase the incidence of foreign-matter aspiration. Impaired swallowing results in coughing or choking on thin liquids. Hoarse, gurgling sounds of the voice may indicate poor oropharynx clearance. Further investigation of airway sounds by auscultation starting at the trachea may aid in the assessment of ineffective swallowing. Dysphagic individuals require meticulous oral care to reduce the risk of aspiration pneumonia.[10]

As individuals lie in bed resting on their back, secretions can collect within the posterior lobes. Static secretions increase the risk of pneumonia development. Even

Table 1
Laboratory values related to the pulmonary system

	Acidosis	Arterial Blood Gases Normal Value	Alkalosis
pH	<7.35	7.35–7.45	>7.45
CO_2, mm Hg	>45	35–45	<35
HCO_3, mEq/L	<22	22–26	>26
O_2, mm Hg	—	80–100	—
Vco_2, mmol/L	Metabolic	24–30	Metabolic
Brain natriuretic peptide (BNP), μg/L		<100	
Serum glucose level, mg/dL		70–110	
Sodium, mg/dL		135–145	
Potassium, mg/dL		3.5–5.0	
Chloride, mg/dL		100–106	
Blood urea nitrogen, mg/dL		8–25	
Creatinine, mg/dL		0.6–1.6	

Data from Venes D, editor. Tabor's cyclopedic medical dictionary. 19th edition. Philadelphia: F.A. Davis; 2001. p. 2448–50; with permission.

healthy older adults' epithelial lining has been found to have an increase in neutrophils and a decrease in macrophages when compared with that of younger adults. Macrophages are effective in eliminating foreign matter and bacteria that reach the lower respiratory tract regions. The decrease in macrophage numbers may place older adults at greater risk for infection within the lungs.[4,11]

Changes in ventilation-perfusion matching and shunting occur with age. This widened alveolar-arterial oxygen gradient does not seem to change the arterial pressures of O_2 or CO_2. Despite this, the older adult may not perceive hypoxic or hypercapnic events in the same way younger adults do, and thus may fail to alert health care personnel. Even though the lack of O_2 or excess CO_2 may cause no apparent distress, abnormal O_2 and CO_2 values are always a cause for concern.[3,4]

Tachypnea is the best indicator of respiratory compromise in the older adult. Febrile presentation cannot be relied on for evidence of infection; only 50% of older adults have a fever with infection.[9,10] Tachypnea with or without activity may not be accompanied with the complaint of dyspnea by the older adult. In fact, older adults experiencing bronchoconstriction may not perceive the symptom even with the occurrence of significant constriction. Tachycardia from any cause can result in hypoxia from poor tissue perfusion.[3,4]

Overall body changes in muscular strength, skeletal structure, and mobility lead to changes in pulmonary function. Musculoskeletal changes alter thoracic mobility. These restrictions have a negative effect on respiration. All older adults have some decrease in thoracic muscular strength and skeletal movement, but some older adults have the added complication of comorbid diseases that increase the effort of breathing. Osteoporosis, spinal column changes such as kyphosis or scoliosis, and traumas to the chest require the individual to exert more effort to breathe in comparison with those unaffected by musculoskeletal disease. Positional support is needed to improve effective respiration. Older adults have improved lung aeration if the head of the bed is elevated at least 15° and as much as 90°. Individuals with chronic obstructive pulmonary disease (COPD) may prefer the orthopnic position.[2,4,12]

Typical Respiratory Diseases in Older Adults

Older adults are at greater risk for pneumonia related to heightened inflammatory activity within the alveoli and bronchiolar spaces. Boyd and Orihuela[13] found increases in inflammatory cells within the lungs and blood of healthy older adults. Although these cells are present, they do not have the effectiveness of fighting infection that occurs in younger adults. It is therefore possible that this contributes to their increased risk of community-acquired pneumonia (CAP). Individuals with COPD have even greater numbers of inflammatory cells than healthy older adults, and their risk of CAP is even greater than that of healthy older adults. Alterations in the pulmonary environment make it clear that pneumonia vaccines are protective in the older adult population.[1]

Individuals who present to the hospital with CAP have signs of acute respiratory infection that include cough, dyspnea, and, possibly, fever. A chest radiograph will indicate an acute infiltrate. Older adults are typically infected with Streptococcus pneumoniae, Haemophilus influenzae, or Klebsiella pneumoniae. Individuals who are admitted to the ICU for CAP have comorbidities. These patients also have fever, tachypnea, tachycardia, and hypotension. A presentation of abnormal chemistries includes arterial pH lower than 7.35, BUN level higher than 64 mg/dL, sodium level less than 130 mEq/L, glucose level greater than 250 mg/dL, Pao_2 less than 60 mm Hg, and Sao_2 less than 90%, as well as a pleural effusion on radiographs. Confusion caused by the altered homeostasis is common.[14]

The nurse should anticipate the treatment of CAP within the ICU to include a macrolide, a fluroquinolone, and a β-lactam. These antibiotics are administered intravenously for 1 week to 10 days. Individuals need to be afebrile and clinically stable before antibiotics are discontinued.[14]

Early signs of COPD are identified as a chronic cough with mucus production, although a cough may occur without noticeable mucus. Forced expiratory volume (FEV) at this time may fall within normal limits. The progression of COPD is apparent with further symptoms of dyspnea and diminishing FEV values. In the elderly, the diagnosis is confounded by the changes of aging that produce decreased FEV and dyspnea. Nonetheless, older adults who have smoked have greater challenges with breathing than do older adults who have quit smoking or have never smoked. Nurses should implement smoking-cessation education for all smokers regardless of the level of disease.[15]

Simple questions designed by the Global Initiative for Chronic Obstructive Lung Disease (GOLD) reveal the toll COPD takes on individuals diagnosed with the disease. Activity levels are graded from 0 to 4, with 0 being breathlessness with strenuous activity and 4 being too breathless to participate in activities of daily living without becoming breathless (**Box 1**). COPD is also quantified from mild to very severe by evaluating FEV after bronchodilator administration. Mild COPD, called GOLD 1, occurs with a FEV of greater than or equal to 80% of the predicted value of expired air for the same age, gender, height, and weight in persons without pulmonary compromise. Very severe COPD trends to such poor FEV that the expired air is less than 30% of the anticipated volume for similar persons without COPD (**Box 2**).[15]

Pulmonary support of individuals with COPD may require the administration of bronchodilators and, at times, corticosteroids. Airways normally dilate with inhalation and constrict with expiration. In the presence of bronchoconstriction and inflammation of COPD, airways become too narrow for effective expiration. β-Agonist bronchodilators exert an effect on β-receptors of the sympathetic nervous system, keeping airways open on expiration. Anticholinergic bronchodilators interfere with the parasympathetic nervous system's stimulus to constrict airways, also keeping airways open with expiration. The β-agonist albuterol and the anticholinergic ipratropium are often combined for the reduction of acute symptoms. Long-acting β-agonists and anticholinergics are prescribed for maintenance care.[15]

Box 1
Modified Medical Research Council (mMRC) questionnaire for assessing the severity of breathlessness

mMRC Grade 0: I only get breathless with strenuous exercise

mMRC Grade 1: I get short of breath when hurrying on the level or walking up a slight hill

mMRC Grade 2: I walk slower than people of the same age on the level because of breathlessness, or I have to stop for breath when walking on my own pace on the level

mMRC Grade 3: I stop for breath after walking about 100 m or after a few minutes on the level

mMRC Grade 4: I am too breathless to leave the house or I am breathless when dressing or undressing

Adapted from Fletcher CM, Elmes PC, Fairbairn MB, et al. The significance of respiratory symptoms and the diagnosis of chronic bronchitis in a working population. Br Med J 1959;2:257–66.

Box 2
Classification of severity of airflow limitation in COPD (based on postbronchodilator FEV_1)

In patients with FEV_1/FVC <0.70
GOLD 1: mild $FEV_1 \geq 80\%$ predicted
GOLD 2: moderate $50\% \leq FEV_1 <80\%$ predicted
GOLD 3: severe $30\% \leq FEV_1 <50\%$ predicted
GOLD 4: very severe $FEV_1 <30\%$ predicted

Abbreviations: COPD, chronic obstructive pulmonary disease; FVC, forced vital capacity; FEV_1, forced expiratory volume in 1 second.
  Reprinted with permission from the Global Strategy for Diagnosis, Management and Prevention of COPD 2011. Available at: http://www.goldcopd.org. © 2011 Global Initiative for Chronic Obstructive Lung Disease, all rights reserved.

Pulmonary Interventions

Oxygen is useful to deter hypoxia in older adults with pulmonary issues. The use of oxygen must be balanced with consideration of the individual's drive to breathe. An older adult with healthy lungs will have a hypercarbic drive to breathe, whereas an older individual with COPD develops a hypoxic drive to breathe. Close observation of respiratory rate and effort on all older adults with oxygen therapy is necessary. Long-term use of oxygen is recommended for those individuals who have a Pao_2 less than 55 mm Hg as evaluated over a 3-week period.[15]

Noninvasive ventilation support has been shown to improve the quality of life for individuals with sleep apnea and COPD. Bilevel positive end-expiratory pressures for inspiration and expiration offer a way to regain adequate oxygenation and relieve hypercarbia in individuals with respiratory failure. The use of noninvasive ventilation requires an individual who is alert, with minimal mucus production, and who is calm enough for application of the facemask.[16] Noninvasive ventilation is as effective for respiratory failure in older adults as endotracheal intubation, but with shorter intensive care and in-hospital stays.[17]

Critical care nurses should encourage teeth brushing and flossing after each meal and bedtime in awake patients. Total-care patients need to have oral care provided at least 4 times a day. Water should be offered to maintain hydration in older adults.[9]

DISCUSSION

Nursing care for older adults requires the knowledge of the physiologic changes in the pulmonary system that result from aging. Bedside nursing care activities that assess and intervene in pulmonary alterations or age-related changes can reduce the number of complications in older adults. Oral care, water supplementation, and body positioning to ease breathing and release musculoskeletal structures may aid older adults in preventing complications attributable to normal aging.[2,3,9]

Further interventions are required for older adults with pulmonary diseases. Nurses can identify individual needs by attending to respiratory rate and effort. Changes in level of consciousness, confusion, agitation, or anxiety should alert the nurse to assess oxygen saturation as well.[17] Nurses should encourage smoking cessation in those older adults who continue to smoke. Even individuals within critical care settings will benefit from ambulation and positional passive exercises to release chest-wall tension.[11,15]

Nurses will continue to care for the older adult in critical settings for the foreseeable future. The population of older adults is increasing. It is important that nurses recognize the difference in expected pulmonary system changes during the aging process, and the pulmonary complications arising from pulmonary disease.

REFERENCES

1. Center for Disease Control and Prevention. Available at: http://www.cdc.gov. Accessed February 28, 2013.
2. Watsford ML, Murphy AJ, Pine MJ. The effects of ageing on respiratory muscle function and performance in older adults. J Sci Med Sport 2006;10:36–44.
3. Martini FH, Nath JL. The respiratory system, fundamentals of anatomy & physiology. 8th edition. San Francisco (CA): Pearson-Benjamin Cummings; 2009. p. 825–73.
4. Zeleznik J. Normative aging of the respiratory system. Clin Geriatr Med 2003;19:1–18.
5. Chang AB, Widdiconbe JG. Cough throughout life: children, adults, and the senile. Pulm Pharmacol Ther 2007;20:371–82.
6. Parkes R. Rate of respiration: the forgotten vital sign. Emerg Nurse 2011;19(2):12–8.
7. Venes D, editor. Taber's cyclopedic medical dictionary. 19th edition. Philadelphia: F.A. Davis Co; 2001. p. 2448–50.
8. Castellanos MR, Szerszen A, Saifan C, et al. Fasting hyperglycemia upon hospital admissions associated with higher pneumonia complication rates among the elderly. Int Arch Med 2010;3(16):1–7.
9. Huber J. Effects of utterance length and vocal loudness on speech breathing. Respir Physiol Neurobiol 2008;164:323–30.
10. Eisenstadt ES. Dysphagia and aspiration pneumonia in older adults. J Am Acad Nurse Pract 2010;22:17–22.
11. Takeshita T, Tomioka M, Shimazaki Y, et al. Microfloral characterization of the tongue coating and associated risk for pneumonia-related health problems in institutionalized older adults. J Am Geriatr Soc 2010;58:1050–7.
12. Ekstrum JA, Black LL, Paschal KA. Effects of a thoracic mobility and respiratory exercise program on pulmonary function and functional capacity in older adults. Phys Occup Ther Geriatr 2009;27(4):310–27.
13. Boyd AR, Orihuela CJ. Dysregulated inflammation as a risk factor for pneumonia in the elderly. Aging Dis 2011;2(6):487–500.
14. Hull CE. Community-acquired pneumonia management guidelines. Clinician Reviews 2007;17(9):28–34.
15. Global Initiative for Chronic Obstructive Lung Disease. Global strategy for the diagnosis, management, and prevention of chronic obstructive pulmonary disease (updated 2013). Available at: www.goldcopd.org. Accessed February 20, 2013.
16. Gursel G, Aydogdu M, Tasyurek S, et al. Factors associated with noninvasive ventilation response in the first day of therapy in patients with hypercapnic respiratory failure. Ann Thorac Med 2012;7(2):92–7.
17. Ramadan FH, El Sohl AA. Comment: respiratory failure in older adults. Respiratory Medicine. 2006; (13616706). pdf 20483752.

Renal Issues in Older Adults in Critical Care

Bryan Boling, RN, CCRN, CEN

KEYWORDS

- Acute kidney injury • Older adults • Critical care • Renal complications

KEY POINTS

- Renal issues are a major source of complications in the intensive care unit.
- Older adults in critical care are at an increased risk for renal complications because of the effects of aging and a higher rate of comorbid conditions that effect kidney function.
- Primary and secondary prevention are the most important management strategies in acute kidney injury.
- Acute kidney injury in older adults in critical care carries a high rate of mortality and morbidity, which increases with the severity of injury.

INTRODUCTION

Renal issues are among the most common complications encountered in critical illness and are known to increase mortality, morbidity, and health care costs.[1-3] As the population ages and medical and surgical treatments for disease become increasingly aggressive, the rates of these complications continue to increase.[3] Older adult patients are at a particular risk for the development of renal problems because of several factors, including the normal effects of aging and a higher rate of comorbid conditions that may affect kidney function.

In recent years, more attention has been paid to the deleterious effects of renal dysfunction at earlier stages of injury. *Acute kidney injury* (AKI) has largely replaced *acute renal failure* as the preferred terminology in referring to renal disease because it highlights the spectrum of injury from oliguria to complete renal collapse. This article describes AKI in critically ill older adults, risk factors for the development of AKI, management techniques, and short- and long-term outcomes in this population.

AKI IN CRITICALLY ILL OLDER ADULTS

One of the challenges in studying the incidence and prevalence of renal dysfunction in critically ill older adults has been the lack of a consensus definition, with various

Disclosures: None.
Cardiothoracic Vascular Intensive Care Unit, University of Kentucky Hospital, 2116 Sage Road, Lexington, KY 40504, USA
E-mail address: bryanboling@uky.edu

studies using widely divergent criteria for renal failure. However, in 2004, the Acute Dialysis Quality Initiative group proposed the RIFLE criteria (Risk, Injury, Failure, Loss, End-stage Renal Disease) for grading and classifying renal injury according to severity.[4] Five levels of renal injury exist under the RIFLE scheme covering the range of AKI, from risk to end-stage renal disease. The RIFLE classification provides specific serum creatinine and urine output criteria for each level (**Table 1**).

Further complicating matters is the ambiguity surrounding the terms *older adult* and *elderly*. Despite the increasing emphasis on geriatric care and research, there is no uniform definition for what constitutes an older adult. Commonly, 60 years of age[5,6] has been used as a lower cutoff for segregating older patients from the rest of the population. However, some have argued that because of the increasing lifespan and improvement in functional health, 70 years of age and older[7] might be a more appropriate definition. Some studies on kidney disease in the elderly define the population even more narrowly, using 80 years of age and older.[6] For the purposes of this article, *older adult* is defined as 60 years of age and older unless otherwise specified.

Despite the challenges presented by ambiguous definitions, recent studies can help to illustrate the incidence and prevalence of AKI in critically ill older adults. A review of the literature concerning studies evaluating the use of RIFLE criteria for epidemiology and outcomes of AKI found that when RIFLE criteria were applied, the incidence of AKI among critically ill patients ranged from 15.4% to 78.3%, with the higher percentages being reported in the higher acuity cohorts.[3] This finding is higher than previously reported using stricter interpretations of acute renal failure, a fact that is not surprising given that the RIFLE criteria purposefully include a wider spectrum of disease than was previously defined.[4] Several studies have identified advanced age as an independent risk factor for the development of AKI.[1,2,8]

RISK FACTORS

Certain anatomic and physiologic changes to the kidney take place as a normal part of the aging process (**Box 1**). As they age, kidneys lose cortical mass, resulting in a loss of 30% to 50% of glomeruli by 70 years of age.[9] This loss, combined with an increase in glomerular sclerosis and a loss of functional renal reserve, results in a marked reduction in the glomerular filtration rate (GFR) and a 50% decrease in renal blood flow.[10] Additionally, there is a significant reduction in the ability to conserve sodium

Table 1 RIFLE criteria		
Stage	**Creatinine Criteria**	**Urine Output Criteria**
Risk	Increase of 1.5–2.0 times baseline (or GFR decrease >25%)	<0.5 mL/kg/h × 6 h
Injury	Increase of 2–3 times baseline (or GFR decrease >50%)	<0.5 mL/kg/h × 12 h
Failure	Increase of >3 times baseline or creatinine value of 4 mg/dL with an acute increase of ≥0.5 mg/dL (or GFR decrease >75%)	<0.3 mg/kg/h × 24 h or anuria × 12 h
Loss	Persistent loss of renal function >4 wk	—
ESKD	ESKD >3 mo	—

Abbreviations: ESKD, end-stage kidney disease; GFR, glomerular filtration rate.

Adapted from Bellomo R, Ronco C, Kellum JA, et al. Acute renal failure - definition, outcome measures, animal models, fluid therapy and information technology needs: the Second International Consensus Conference of the Acute Dialysis Quality Initiative (ADQI) Group. Crit Care 2004;8(4):R206.

Box 1
Anatomic and physiologic changes to the kidney associated with aging

Anatomic Changes

- Decrease in renal mass
- Reduction in number of functional glomeruli
- Glomerular hypertrophy and sclerosis

Physiologic Changes

- Decrease in glomerular filtration rate
- Decrease in renal blood flow
- Decrease in ability to concentrate urine and conserve water

---

and concentrate urine,[11] placing older patients at an increased risk for hypovolemia and the development of renal hypoperfusion.

An additional consequence of aging is the decrease in lean body mass, resulting in alterations of cellular hydration and total body water distribution.[5] This result seems to decrease the amount of intracellular water while increasing the amount of extracellular water during periods of stress, such as critical illness. Hence, a state of cellular dehydration is created, which has particularly important implications for the use of nephrotoxic agents, such as nonsteroidal antiinflammatory drugs (NSAIDs), certain antibiotics, and radiocontrast dye, causing an artificial extracellular dilution of drugs that may falsely decrease plasma levels while simultaneously causing an increase in the concentration of drug within the cell, leading to toxicities.[5] Not only is this important to remember during the care of critically ill older patients but this may also affect the baseline kidney function if patients are taking large doses of NSAIDs or other potentially nephrotoxic drugs chronically.

Beyond the normal effects of aging, older adults have a greatly increased incidence of comorbid conditions that affect renal function, such as cardiovascular disease, diabetes, and urinary obstruction.[7] Given the increased incidence of cardiovascular disease among older adults, the possibility of cardiorenal syndrome, a clinical condition whereby heart failure may precipitate renal failure, should not be ignored.[12] Scrutinio and colleagues[12] found that heart failure in combination with renal failure significantly increased the risk for death or a need for urgent heart transplantation. Ruggenenti and colleagues[13] found a GFR decline among patients with diabetes to proceed at an average rate of 3 mL/min/1.73^2/y, more than triple the rate among nondiabetics. This decline in GFR weakens the kidneys over time, predisposing them to chronic kidney disease and AKI.[13] Finally, Feest and colleagues[14] found that 35% of cases of AKI in older men were caused by postrenal obstruction and could be directly attributable to benign prostatic hyperplasia.

Many older patients in the intensive care unit (ICU) undergo surgical procedures of various types. Between 7% and 31% of all patients undergoing surgery will develop AKI, depending on the specific type of surgery and the comorbidities associated with the patients.[15] This risk can be mitigated in many cases by identifying patients who are at an increased risk preoperatively, avoiding nephrotoxic agents if possible, and maintaining adequate volume status throughout the perioperative period.[15]

Finally, sepsis represents one of the largest risk factors for the development of AKI among all critically ill patients. Although septic AKI has not been studied extensively, the general risk among older adults for infection, combined with additional AKI risk factors in this population, may put elderly ICU patients at an increased risk. Bagshaw and colleagues[16] determined sepsis to be the primary cause of AKI in 47.5% of cases.

MANAGEMENT

Management strategies for AKI in older adults do not differ from those for the general population.[6] The best management strategy remains the prevention of the initial renal insult. If AKI does develop, prevention strategies may be used to limit the progression. This limitation is crucial because outcomes worsen as the degree of renal failure increases.[3] A list of prevention strategies is provided in **Box 2**. Maintenance of fluid and electrolyte balance is particularly important in this population given the reduction in sodium conservation and increased risk of hypovolemia among older patients.[11] It is also critical to dose drugs according to renal function when appropriate[6]; consultation with a critical care pharmacist may be useful in these cases.

If prevention and limitation strategies are unsuccessful, more aggressive therapy is warranted. Although patients requiring use of renal replacement therapy (RRT) have been shown to have an increased mortality over patients who do not,[3] most studies do not specifically identify RRT usage as an independent risk factor for mortality.[1,2,8] Mortality increases with the degree of renal failure,[3] so it is possible that the increased mortality among patients undergoing RRT is the result of the increased severity of renal disease necessitating the RRT rather than the RRT itself. RRT in older patients has been shown to be safe and well tolerated and should be initiated if needed to adequately control fluid and electrolyte balance.[7]

OUTCOMES

In a study of 19,982 hospitalized adults, Chertow and colleagues[1] found that even a modest increase in serum creatinine of 0.3 mg/dL or greater carried a 6.6-fold increase in mortality (95% confidence interval 5.0–8.7) in older patients. Uchino and colleagues[2] found an overall in-hospital mortality rate of 60.3%, with 52.0% of patients dying while still in the ICU. This finding was significantly larger than the predicted mortality rate of 45.6%, indicating that AKI may increase mortality beyond what would be expected based on the overall degree of illness. Advanced age has been repeatedly identified as an independent risk factor for in-hospital mortality in AKI.[1,2,8] The severity of AKI and the requirement of RRT both have been shown to increase mortality.[3]

Box 2
Prevention and limitation of AKI in critically ill older adults

- Optimize hemodynamics, including preload, cardiac output, and mean arterial pressure
- Optimize fluid volume status
- Limit fluid volume loss
- Limit use of nephrotoxic drugs, consult pharmacy for renal dosing when appropriate
- Use judicious use of contrast medium; consider use of bicarbonate and/or N-acetylcysteine when appropriate
- Maintain alertness for signs and symptoms of sepsis; treat aggressively with appropriate antibiotics

Adapted from Chronopoulos A, Rosner MH, Cruz DN, et al. Acute kidney injury in elderly intensive care patients: a review. Intensive Care Med 2010;36(9):1459; with permission.

AKI also carries an increase in morbidity and the associated costs. Patients with AKI have an increased length of stay of between 3.5 and 9.0 days and an increased cost of between $5000 and $33,000 per hospitalization, depending on the severity.[1] In addition to these short-term complications, AKI survivors may have significant long-term effects, with nearly 50% of patients requiring extensive care following discharge, either through home health or inpatient care in an extended-care facility.[17] In one recent study of the long-term outcomes of critically ill patients with AKI, approximately 30% failed to regain normal renal function by 90 days following discharge and 22% still required hemodialysis 1 year later.[18] A meta-analysis by Schmitt and colleagues[19] found that 31.3% of elderly patients failed to recover kidney function following discharge, compared with 26.0% of younger patients.

SUMMARY

Renal complications are commonly seen in the care of critically ill patients. Several factors increase the risk of critically ill older patients. Normal aging combined with higher rates of other chronic diseases already predispose older patients to the development of AKI. When the stresses of critical illness are factored in, the risk increases even greater. AKI is a progressive spectrum of renal dysfunction that increases mortality and morbidity. Prevention is the best management strategy, although the limitation of progression and aggressive RRT may be of value in optimizing patient outcomes.

REFERENCES

1. Chertow GM, Burdick E, Honour M, et al. Acute kidney injury, mortality, length of stay, and costs in hospitalized patients. J Am Soc Nephrol 2005;16(11):3365–70.
2. Uchino S, Kellum JA, Bellomo R, et al. Acute renal failure in critically ill patients: a multinational, multicenter study. JAMA 2005;294(7):813–8.
3. Hoste EA, Kellum JA. Acute kidney injury: epidemiology and diagnostic criteria. Curr Opin Crit Care 2006;12(6):531–7.
4. Bellomo R, Ronco C, Kellum JA, et al. Acute renal failure - definition, outcome measures, animal models, fluid therapy and information technology needs: the Second International Consensus Conference of the Acute Dialysis Quality Initiative (ADQI) Group. Crit Care 2004;8(4):R204–12.
5. Ritz P. Chronic cellular dehydration in the aged patient. J Gerontol A Biol Sci Med Sci 2001;56(6):M349–52.
6. Chronopoulos A, Rosner MH, Cruz DN, et al. Acute kidney injury in elderly intensive care patients: a review. Intensive Care Med 2010;36(9):1454–64.
7. Pascual J, Liano F, Ortuno J. The elderly patient with acute renal failure. J Am Soc Nephrol 1995;6(2):144–53.
8. de Mendonca A, Vincent JL, Suter PM, et al. Acute renal failure in the ICU: risk factors and outcome evaluated by the SOFA score. Intensive Care Med 2000; 26(7):915–21.
9. Goyal VK. Changes with age in the human kidney. Exp Gerontol 1982;17(5):321–31.
10. Esposito C, Plati A, Mazzullo T, et al. Renal function and functional reserve in healthy elderly individuals. J Nephrol 2007;20(5):617–25.
11. Rowe JW, Shock NW, DeFronzo RA. The influence of age on the renal response to water deprivation in man. Nephron 1976;17(4):270–8.
12. Scrutinio D, Passantino A, Santoro D, et al. The cardiorenal anaemia syndrome in systolic heart failure: prevalence, clinical correlates, and long-term survival. Eur J Heart Fail 2011;13(1):61–7.

13. Ruggenenti P, Porrini EL, Gaspari F, et al. Glomerular hyperfiltration and renal disease progression in type 2 diabetes. Diabetes Care 2012;35(10):2061–8.

14. Feest TG, Round A, Hamad S. Incidence of severe acute renal failure in adults: results of a community based study. BMJ 1993;306(6876):481–3.

15. Noor S, Usmani A. Postoperative renal failure. Clin Geriatr Med 2008;24(4): 721–9, ix.

16. Bagshaw SM, Uchino S, Bellomo R, et al. Septic acute kidney injury in critically ill patients: clinical characteristics and outcomes. Clin J Am Soc Nephrol 2007;2(3): 431–9.

17. Fischer MJ, Brimhall BB, Parikh CR. Uncomplicated acute renal failure and posthospital care: a not so uncomplicated illness. Am J Nephrol 2008;28(3):523–30.

18. Bagshaw SM, Laupland KB, Doig CJ, et al. Prognosis for long-term survival and renal recovery in critically ill patients with severe acute renal failure: a population-based study. Crit Care 2005;9(6):R700–9.

19. Schmitt R, Coca S, Kanbay M, et al. Recovery of kidney function after acute kidney injury in the elderly: a systematic review and meta-analysis. Am J Kidney Dis 2008;52(2):262–71.

Aging Muscles and Joints
Mobilization

Helen W. Lach, PhD, RN, GCNS-BC*, Rebecca A. Lorenz, PhD, RN,
Kristine M. L'Ecuyer, PhD(c), RN, CCNS, CNL

KEYWORDS

- Aging • Critical care • Mobilization • Mobility programs

KEY POINTS

- Aging causes older adults to quickly experience a decline in muscle mass, muscle strength, and joint mobility, with immobilization that is common in critical illness.
- Early and progressive mobilization can reduce these losses, but may be missed in many patients.
- Nearly all older patients can participate in progressive mobility programs tailored to their status.
- Development of protocols with the intensive care unit team promotes consistent implementation of mobilization in older patients.

INTRODUCTION

The US Public Health Service first reported the negative effects of immobilization more than 40 years ago.[1] Following that report, the detrimental effect of bed rest during hospitalization on mobilization was summarized in the *American Journal of Nursing*.[2] Elderly individuals whose mobility is restricted because of acute illness have the greatest risk of deconditioning. Absolute bed rest accelerates the loss of muscle mass and strength by about 1.5% per day.[3]

The effect of hospitalization on mobility was further elucidated by a small study, which explored the functioning of patients on a daily basis.[4] The researchers found that older patients experience new and worsened functional impairment as early as the second day of hospitalization. It has been shown that patients in acute care settings only perform about 5 minutes (standard deviation 9.2) of physical activity in a 24-hour period,[5,6] which places them at high risk for deterioration in functional ability.[7,8]

There is no funding support for this article.
The authors have nothing to disclose.
Saint Louis University School of Nursing, 3525 Caroline Mall, St Louis, MO 63104, USA
* Corresponding author.
E-mail address: lachh@slu.edu

Other researchers have replicated and extended the findings of this landmark study by examining the effects of functional decline during and after discharge from the hospital. Of the 30% to 35% of older patients who experienced this decline, more than half had died or had a new impairment.[9,10] Those who had the greatest functional decline during hospitalization were most likely to be admitted to a nursing home.[11] Overall, immobility and functional decline have far-reaching effects for older patients.

Recent studies have demonstrated improved functional outcomes, improved morbidity, and lower overall hospital costs for patients in the intensive care unit (ICU) who receive early mobilization.[12–16] The literature identifies that some mobilization is possible for almost every patient, based on the individual's medical condition as well as devices and equipment.[17] With the large body of evidence supporting it, and the potential negative effects of immobility, early progressive mobility should be a standard of care for critically ill older adults.[18] This article addresses aging changes and other factors that affect muscles and joints, and the nursing implications for mobilization of critically ill older patients.

AGING MUSCLES

In the older adult population, skeletal muscle changes in acute care are related to aging, inactivity, underlying medical conditions, poor nutritional status, and hormonal changes. The human body contains more than 400 skeletal muscles, which make up 30% to 40% of the total body weight. It is well established that aging is associated with a reduction in skeletal muscle mass and strength called sarcopenia, even in healthy older adults.[19] A recent study showed that the prevalence of low muscle mass increases with aging from 8.9% in the 76- to 80-year age group to 10.9% in 86- to 95-year age group.[20] The impact of the aging process on skeletal muscles and joints can have a profound effect on the functionality of an individual, especially when coupled with sedentary behavior. Reduced skeletal muscle mass can adversely affect balance and has been associated with functional decline, particularly in older women.[21]

Age-related skeletal muscle changes vary among muscle groups and for different muscle fiber types, and do not affect all muscles equally.[22] It has been reported that aging muscle shows a reduction in the number and total size of fast-twitch muscle fibers and a reduction in number of slow-twitch muscle fibers.[23] A study by Poggi and colleagues[24] showed a predominance of type I fibers in aging muscles, and suggested that this could be secondary to selective atrophy of type II fibers or a conversion of type II to type I fibers. In comparison with non–weight-bearing muscles, weight-bearing muscles having a higher proportion of type II fibers showed marked atrophy.[25]

Numerous age-related changes in other subsystems, such as reductions in neuromuscular innervation, insulin activity, estrogen, testosterone, and growth hormone levels, as well as weight loss, protein deficiency, and physical inactivity, can contribute to loss of muscle mass and strength in older people.[26] Taken together, these changes lead older adults to have a high risk for weakness and muscle loss from lack of physical activity and immobility. For example, an older person may lose up to 2 lb ($\sim$ 1 kg) of leg muscle from 10 days of bed rest,[27] which is accompanied by loss of aerobic capacity and strength.

AGING JOINTS

The synovial joint (or movable joint) is a critically important biomechanical structure for mobilization, with several key components contributing to overall function. Muscles that envelop the joint provide stability and strength along with ligaments and tendons, which provide movement and stability. Articular cartilage reduces the friction in the articulating surfaces that participate in weight bearing. The synovial membrane secretes synovial fluid that lubricates the joint space. Each of these components undergoes age-related changes that make the joint more susceptible to age-related diseases and injury,[28] such as arthritis. Joint contractures having an impact on function have been shown to develop with immobilization in critically ill patients, affecting ambulation even after discharge.[29] Decreased muscle strength may play a significant role in promoting joint injury because the stabilizing function of the muscles in joint biomechanics is compromised.[30]

OTHER FACTORS AFFECTING MOBILIZATION OF OLDER CRITICALLY ILL PATIENTS

In addition to aging changes, a variety of other factors influence mobility and functional decline in critically ill patients (**Table 1**). These factors include medical conditions, nutrition, treatment devices and equipment, restraints, and staff priorities. Chronic conditions common among older adults may enhance problems related to skeletal muscles in critical illness. For example, heart failure causes significant changes in skeletal muscle mitochondria and capillary distribution, which affect the oxidative capacity of working muscle.[31] Chronic renal failure affects the muscle energy metabolism by decreasing the mitochondrial enzymatic activity.[32] Conditions directly affecting muscles and joints, such as arthritis or Parkinson disease, may affect mobilization, resulting in pain, weakness, muscle spasticity, and other effects. Prior medical conditions can be identified in the patient's history.

Inadequate dietary protein intake by older adults has been associated with a loss of skeletal muscle mass, and may affect mobilization. Even healthy older adults do not often get enough dietary protein to meet daily recommendations,[33] and protein-calorie supplementation has shown to be helpful in gaining strength and muscle mass.[34] It is highly likely that critically ill older people do not have adequate protein intake, and more research is needed to determine optimal nutritional support for this group.[35] Inadequate dietary intake could further affect muscles, in addition to immobility.

Table 1
Factors that contribute to immobility in the older adult in critical care settings

Factors Related to Sensation	Factors Related to Physiologic Status	Factors Related to Comorbidities	Factors Related to Psychological Status	Factors Related to Staff
Cognition	Age-related muscle	Traumas	Anxiety	Priority of
Sedation	weakness	Surgery	Fear	mobilization
Analgesia	Pain or discomfort	Obesity	Emotional status	Concerns about
Altered sleep	Metabolism	Burns		equipment and
Delirium	Nutrition and	Malnourishment		patient status
	hydration	Ventilation		Staffing
	Neurologic stability	Indwelling catheters		Interdisciplinary
	Respiratory	Restraints		team support
	stability	Endotracheal tubes		
	Cardiovascular	Assist devices		
	stability	Other medical		
	Vital signs	devices		
	Hemodynamic	Chronic conditions		
	status	affecting muscles		
		and joints		

Patient conditions that necessitate critical care result in significant use of medical devices, lines, and treatments that make mobilization challenging. Nurses have legitimate concerns about dislodging equipment and accidents that may affect patients. However, successful mobilization programs have been reported for even the most challenging patients.[36] Freeman and Maley[13] reported on methods for mobilizing patients with mechanical circulatory support devices. Other reports discuss patients with burns,[37] abdominal surgery,[38] continuous renal replacement therapy,[39] and neurologic disorders.[40] Often mobilization of these complex patients requires several people to assist in their management and safely perform progressive mobilization.

Because mobility and ambulation can improve outcomes and decrease costs for critically ill older adults, mobility must be a priority of care. However, historically mobility and ambulation have been a low priority for the health care team. For example, studies on the frequency of physical therapy in ICUs, particularly patients with mechanical ventilation, have found that physical therapy is used on an inconsistent basis, or very infrequently.[15,41,42]

MOBILIZATION OF CRITICALLY ILL OLDER PATIENTS

Mobilization can be performed to some degree on every patient. The nature of critical illnesses and the ICU environment present potential barriers to mobility and the implementation of early ambulation for the older adult in critical care settings. Some of these barriers include issues related to time, safety, obesity, lack of knowledge, lack of a team approach, resources, and a lack of a climate conducive to early mobility.[15,43,44] Age contributes to these challenges, as older patients have more comorbidities, weakness, and aging changes that make them more susceptible to the effects of their acute illness. Likewise, however, older patients may benefit the most from early mobilization because recovery from side effects of immobility can be lengthy, and many older adults never return to their pre-illness level of functioning.[45]

Conventional interventions related to mobility for the ICU patient center on semirecumbent positioning, turning every 2 hours, range of motion, sitting up in bed, sitting at the edge of bed to dangle lower extremities, standing at the bedside transferring to a bedside chair, and ultimately ambulating in a hallway. The extent and frequency to which these interventions are implemented in ICUs has not been well documented. However, the trend is moving toward early and consistent mobilization as the standard of care,[45] and early mobility programs can successfully be implemented. Components of, and issues with, mobility programs are discussed here.

Program Components

In an effort to increase attention regarding the issue of early mobility, protocols, algorithms, care bundles, checklists, and order sets have been developed to assist health care teams to prioritize mobility. A Delphi study was recently completed in an attempt to formulate evidence-based practice guidelines related to early physical activity and mobilization of critically ill patients.[46] The investigators conducted a thorough review of the current literature, and drafted algorithm statements related to assessment and treatment of critically ill patients in the ICU. Experts from around the world collaborated in the creation of a clinical management algorithm for the mobilization of adult patients in the ICU. The experts listed the following 4 factors as essential to any mobilization plan: (1) inclusion of a mobilization plan for every patient admitted to an ICU, (2) individual patient assessment, (3) clinician's judgment, and (4) interprofessional consultation.

Several examples of early mobility programs for ICU patients have recently been published.[43,46–49] Some mobility programs are nurse driven,[48] whereas others include both nursing and physical therapy goals and interventions.[50] However, all of these programs emphasize the integration of evidence-based guidelines that are meaningful and individualized to the patient's physiologic status and mobility potential. Themes found across these mobility programs are patient assessment, identification of patient readiness to participate in a mobility program, initiation of core interventions, and teamwork. These themes should be maintained in any new mobility programs for critically ill older adults.

Patient Assessment

Patient assessment is a strong component of all mobility programs. Patients should be assessed early, and routinely, for establishment of medical stability and to guide the timing of the initiation and progression of mobility initiatives. Some programs start the patient on a progressive mobility algorithm as early as 8 hours after admission to the ICU,[51] although turning should begin immediately. Most programs call for at least daily assessment of mobility levels. All programs advocate for specific assessment of factors that facilitate or impede mobility. These factors can be viewed as modifiable and nonmodifiable,[43] to help guide nursing assessment, patient selection, and implementation of mobility programs. Modifiable factors might be considerations such as sedation, delirium, sleep, pain, and respiratory/ventilator status.

Mobility programs must have clear guidelines and specific inclusion criteria for patient selection and initiation of mobility programs (**Table 2**). The pulmonary and cardiac systems are assessed for sufficient reserve, and the neurologic system, hematologic system, and other related factors are evaluated for favorability of conditions.[16,36,52] Beyond physiologic factors, readiness for initiation of a mobility program may include an assessment of the patient's ability to raise each leg against gravity in the supine position, ability to sit on the side of the bed with minimal support, standing at the bedside with walker and assistance, ability to shift weight laterally with walker and assistance, ability to take steps in place with walker and assistance, and progressive walking with walker and assistance.[52]

The mobility team monitors the patient for responses that might indicate that the patient is not tolerating the intervention. As with other treatments in older adults, the approach is to proceed slowly, as adjustment to changes in position or activity may take longer than in younger patients. The following may indicate the need for a delay in or termination of the intervention[16,46,52]:

1. Chest pain and electrocardiographic changes, ectopic beats, or arrhythmias
2. Increase or decrease in heart rate (10–20 beats above resting baseline)
3. Changes in blood pressure (>170 mm Hg systolic, or >110 mm Hg diastolic, or a drop of >10 mm Hg systolic)
4. Dizziness, light-headedness, diaphoresis, pallor, pain, discomfort, fatigue
5. Spo_2 (oxygen saturation) less than 92%, or signs of respiratory distress such as dyspnea or cyanosis

Core Interventions

Mobility programs should be interdisciplinary and should include respiratory therapy, nursing, and physical therapy. Respiratory therapists are vital, particularly for ventilated patients, to assess and monitor the airway and oxygen therapies. Nursing roles include assessment and management of level of consciousness (delirium, sedation, and sleep), pain, psychological issues, and the patient's physiologic readiness and tolerance to therapy. Physical therapy includes assistance with range of motion and strengthening exercises, bed mobility exercises and positioning, transfer and gait

Table 2
Criteria for patient selection for mobilization

Neurologic	Awake, alert Normalized intracranial pressure Able to respond and follow verbal commands Cooperation
Respiratory	Fio_2 <50%, PEEP <8 mm Hg Mechanical ventilation able to be maintained during activity Respiratory rate <30 breaths/min Spo_2 >90% Minimal secretions Appropriate RSBI
Cardiovascular	Hemodynamic stability: blood pressure <20% variability recently No angina Heart rate <130 beats/min; resting heart rate <50% age-predicted maximal heart rate ECG normal: no evidence of MI or arrhythmia No vasopressors
Hematologic	Hemoglobin stable and >7 g/dL Platelet count stable and >20,000 cells/mm³ White cell count 4300–10,800 cells/mm³
Other	Body temperature <38 C Acceptable pain, fatigue, emotional status No orthopedic contraindications Medically stable if DVT or PE Excessive weight able to be safely managed Safe environment Adequate staffing and expertise Patient consent

Abbreviations: DVT, deep venous thrombosis; ECG, electrocardiogram; Fio_2, fraction of inspired oxygen; MI, myocardial infarction; PE, pulmonary embolism; PEEP, positive end-expiratory pressure; RSBI, rapid shallow breathing index; Spo_2, oxygen saturation.
    Data from Refs.[16,18,52]

training, and ambulating in hallways. The goal of all mobility programs is to improve muscle strength, endurance, and function.[52]

Most programs advocate stratification of patients into categories based on the patients' physiologic status. For example, in the Delphi study by Hanekom and colleagues[46] the research group designed 3 algorithms based on 3 patient categories: category A patients are unconscious; category B patients are awake, physiologically stable, and may be on a ventilator; category C patients are deconditioned patients who have been immobile because of a physiologic instability. In addition, category C patients may still be on a ventilator. Mobility interventions for category A patients include semirecumbent positioning with the head of the bed at 30° to 45° or higher, regular position changes, and passive movements of the upper and lower extremity joints daily. Category B patients should progress from lying to sitting to standing, transferring to a chair, walking with assistance, walking independently, and finally climbing stairs. Upper and lower limb-strengthening exercises can also be considered. The trunk, upper limbs, and lower limbs are targeted for strengthening and endurance for category C patients, including low-resistance multiple repetitions, with exercise occurring once daily and progressing to twice daily. Other strategies that might be implemented in these categories are breathing exercises and assisted coughing to increase inspiratory volume and increase pulmonary muscle function, muscle stretching and neuromuscular electrical stimulation to prevent muscle atrophy, cycling pedals in bed, lateral rotation beds, stepping in place, and chair exercises.[36,47]

SUMMARY

Older adults are at risk for significant functional decline from immobility during critical illnesses, but early mobilization and mobility programs can improve outcomes for these vulnerable patients. As aging changes in the muscles and joints increase weakness and response to immobility among older patients, these patients can benefit greatly from nursing interventions to keep them moving and to encourage them to rise from bed as soon as possible. Research and model programs have identified key components to successful mobilization of critically ill patients that can be implemented in all ICUs.

REFERENCES

1. Graf C. Functional decline in hospitalized older adults. Am J Nurs 2006;106: 58–67 [quiz: 67–8].
2. Olson EV, Johnson BJ, Thompson LF. The hazards of immobility. 1967. Am J Nurs 1990;90:43–8.
3. Topp R, Ditmyer M, King K, et al. The effect of bed rest and potential of prehabilitation on patients in the intensive care unit. AACN Clin Issues 2002;13: 263–76.
4. Hirsch CH, Sommers L, Olsen A, et al. The natural history of functional morbidity in hospitalized older patients. J Am Geriatr Soc 1990;38:1296–303.
5. Boltz M, Resnick B, Capezuti E, et al. Functional decline in hospitalized older adults: can nursing make a difference? Geriatr Nurs 2012;33:272–9.
6. Boltz M, Resnick B, Galik E. Function and physical activity across settings: where are we and where do we need to go? Gerontologist 2010;50(S1):297.
7. Hennessy D, Juzwishin K, Yergens D, et al. Outcomes of elderly survivors of intensive care: a review of the literature. Chest 2005;127:1764–74.
8. Wunsch H, Guerra C, Barnato AE, et al. Three-year outcomes for Medicare beneficiaries who survive intensive care. J Am Med Assoc 2010;303:849–56.
9. Landefeld CS, Palmer RM, Kresevic DM, et al. A randomized trial of care in a hospital medical unit especially designed to improve the functional outcomes of acutely ill older patients. N Engl J Med 1995;332:1338–44.
10. Sager MA, Franke T, Inouye SK, et al. Functional outcomes of acute medical illness and hospitalization in older persons. Arch Intern Med 1996;156:645–52.
11. Rudberg MA, Sager MA, Zhang J. Risk factors for nursing home use after hospitalization for medical illness. J Gerontol A Biol Sci Med Sci 1996;51: M189–94.
12. Bailey P, Thomsen GE, Spuhler VJ, et al. Early activity is feasible and safe in respiratory failure patients. Crit Care Med 2007;35:139–45.
13. Freeman R, Maley K. Mobilization of intensive care cardiac surgery patients on mechanical circulatory support. Crit Care Nurs Q 2013;36:73–88.
14. Gillick BT, Marshall WJ, Rheault W, et al. Mobility criteria for upright sitting with patients in the neuro/trauma intensive care unit: an analysis of length of stay and functional outcomes. Neurohospitalist 2011;1:172–7.
15. Morris PE, Herridge MS. Early intensive care unit mobility: future directions. Crit Care Clin 2007;23:97–110.

16. Ronnebaum JA, Weir JP, Hilsabeck TA. Earlier mobilization decreases the length of stay in the intensive care unit. J Acute Care Phys Ther 2012;3:204–10.

17. Vollman KM. Introduction to progressive mobility. Crit Care Nurse 2010;30:S3–5.

18. Rukstele CD, Gagnon MM. Making strides in preventing ICU-acquired weakness: involving family in early progressive mobility. Crit Care Nurs Q 2013;36: 141–7.

19. Doherty TJ. Invited review: aging and sarcopenia. J Appl Phys 2003;95: 1717–27.

20. Gillette-Guyonnet S, Nourhashemi F, Andrieu S, et al. Body composition in French women 75+ years of age: the EPIDOS study. Mech Ageing Dev 2003; 124:311–6.

21. Rantanen T, Guralnik JM, Leveille S, et al. Racial differences in muscle strength in disabled older women. J Gerontol A Biol Sci Med Sci 1998;53:B355–61.

22. Nikolic M, Malnar-Dragojevic D, Bobinac D, et al. Age-related skeletal muscle atrophy in humans: an immunohistochemical and morphometric study. Coll Antropol 2001;25:545–53.

23. Kamel HK, Maas D, Duthie EH. Role of hormones in the pathogenesis and management of sarcopenia. Drugs Aging 2002;19:865–77.

24. Poggi P, Marchetti C, Scelsi R. Automatic morphometric analysis of skeletal muscle fibers in the aging man. Anat Rec 1987;217:30–4.

25. Holloszy JO, Chen M, Cartee GD, et al. Skeletal muscle atrophy in old rats: differential changes in the three fiber types. Mech Ageing Dev 1991;60: 199–213.

26. Hooyman N, Kiyak HA. Social gerontology: a multidisciplinary perspective. 9th edition. Boston, MA: Pearson; 2012.

27. Kortebein P, Symons TB, Ferrando A, et al. Functional impact of 10 days of bed rest in healthy older adults. J Gerontol A Biol Sci Med Sci 2008;63:1076–81.

28. Pacifici M, Koyama E, Iwamoto M. Mechanisms of synovial joint and articular cartilage formation: recent advances, but many lingering mysteries. Birth Defects Res C Embryo Today 2005;75:237–48.

29. Clavet H, Hebert PC, Fergusson DA, et al. Joint contractures in the intensive care unit: association with resource utilization and ambulatory status at discharge. Disabil Rehabil 2011;33:105–12.

30. Brandt KD. Putting some muscle into osteoarthritis. Ann Intern Med 1997;127: 154–6.

31. Drexler H, Riede U, Munzel T, et al. Alterations of skeletal muscle in chronic heart failure. Circulation 1992;85:1751–9.

32. Conjard A, Ferrier B, Martin M, et al. Effects of chronic renal failure on enzymes of energy metabolism in individual human muscle fibers. J Am Soc Nephrol 1995;6:68–74.

33. Campbell WW, Trappe TA, Wolfe RR, et al. The recommended dietary allowance for protein may not be adequate for older people to maintain skeletal muscle. J Gerontol A Biol Sci Med Sci 2001;56:M373–80.

34. Evans WJ. Protein nutrition and resistance exercise. Can J Appl Physiol 2001; 26(Suppl):S141–52.

35. Cherry-Bukowiec JR. Optimizing nutrition therapy to enhance mobility in critically ill patients. Crit Care Nurs Q 2013;36:28–36.

36. Gosselink R, Bott J, Johnson M, et al. Physiotherapy for adult patients with critical illness: recommendations of the European Respiratory Society and European Society of Intensive Care Medicine task force on physiotherapy for critically ill patients. Intensive Care Med 2008;34:1188–99.

37. Taylor S, Manning S, Quarles J. A multidisciplinary approach to early mobilization of patients with burns. Crit Care Nurs Q 2013;36:56–62.
38. Havey R, Herriman E, O'Brien D. Guarding the gut: early mobility after abdominal surgery. Crit Care Nurs Q 2013;36:63–72.
39. Talley CL, Wonnacott RO, Schuette JK, et al. Extending the benefits of early mobility to critically ill patients undergoing continuous renal replacement therapy: the Michigan experience. Crit Care Nurs Q 2013;36:89–100.
40. Kocan MJ, Lietz H. Special considerations for mobilizing patients in the neuro-intensive care unit. Crit Care Nurs Q 2013;36:50–5.
41. Bahadur K, Jones G, Ntoumenopoulos G. An observational study of sitting out of bed in tracheostomised patients in the intensive care unit. Physiotherapy 2008; 94:300–5.
42. Needham M. Mobilizing patients in the intensive care unit: improving neuromuscular weakness and physical function. J Am Med Assoc 2008;300:1685–90.
43. Hopkins RO. Strategies for promoting early activity in critically ill mechanically ventilated patients. AACN Adv Crit Care 2009;20:277–89.
44. Truong AD, Fan E, Brower RG, et al. Bench-to-bedside review: mobilizing patients in the intensive care unit—from pathophysiology to clinical trials. Crit Care 2009;13:216.
45. D'Ambruoso S, Cadogan M. Recognizing hospital-acquired disability among older adults. J Gerontol Nurs 2012;38:12–5.
46. Hanekom S, Gosselink R, Dean E, et al. The development of a clinical management algorithm for early physical activity and mobilization of critically ill patients: synthesis of evidence and expert opinion and its translation into practice. Clin Rehabil 2011;25:771–87.
47. Dammeyer J, Dickinson S, Packard D, et al. Building a protocol to guide mobility in the ICU. Crit Care Nurs Q 2013;36:37–49.
48. Drolet A, Dejuilio P, Harkless S, et al. Move to improve: the feasibility of using an early mobility protocol to increase ambulation in the intensive and intermediate care settings. Phys Ther 2013;93:197–207.
49. Perme C, Chandrashekar R. Early mobility and walking program for patients in intensive care units: creating a standard of care. Am J Crit Care 2009;18: 212–21.
50. Dammeyer JA, Baldwin N, Packard D, et al. Mobilizing outcomes: implementation of a nurse-led multidisciplinary mobility program. Crit Care Nurs Q 2013;36: 109–19.
51. Bassett RD, Vollman KM, Brandwene L, et al. Integrating a multidisciplinary mobility programme into intensive care practice (IMMPTP): a multicentre collaborative. Intensive Crit Care Nurs 2012;28:88–97.
52. Perme C, Chandrashekar RK. Managing the patient on mechanical ventilation in ICU: early mobility and walking program. Acute Care Perspectives 2008;17: 10–5.

Psychiatric Disorders Impacting Critical Illness

Laura M. Struble, PhD, RN, GNP-BC[a],*,
Barbara J. Sullivan, PhD, RN, APRN-BC, NP[a],
Laurie S. Hartman, DNP, RN, ACNP-BC[b]

KEYWORDS

- Psychiatric disorders • Older adults • Critical care • Medical illness

KEY POINTS

- Complications from psychiatric disorders along with medical disorders treated in critical care are often reciprocally complicating.
- Psychiatric patients' stability may be challenged by the speed, chaos, and physical intrusions imposed by medical treatments in a medical emergency department or intensive care unit (ICU).
- Newly stabilized medical/surgical ICU patients may become quickly destabilized by the their paranoid delusions brought on by unanticipated medication interactions.
- Treatment of each is complex; treatment of both simultaneously is an art.
- Prehospitalization preparation, family communication, team collaboration, and a calm focus on the patients' mental status are essential to minimizing additional stress for all involved.
- Patients' treatment can be seriously compromised after discharge if families do not consider themselves allies in the treatment.

INTRODUCTION

More than 40% of older adults, aged 65 years and older, will have a major psychiatric illness by the year 2030.[1] This heterogeneous group has an extreme range of symptoms and illness severity. Although many older patients develop a psychiatric disorder in their teens or young adulthood, some older adults do not experience their first symptoms until after the age of 65 years. As older adults with psychiatric disorders face the challenges of aging, they also have premature mortality and poor outcomes

The authors have nothing to disclose.
[a] Division of Acute, Critical and Long-Term Care, University of Michigan School of Nursing, 400 North Ingalls Building, Ann Arbor, MI 48109, USA; [b] University of Michigan Hospitals and Health System, University of Michigan School of Nursing, 400 North Ingalls Building, Ann Arbor, MI 48109, USA
* Corresponding author. Division of Acute, Critical and Long-Term Care, University of Michigan School of Nursing, 400 North Ingalls Building, Ann Arbor, MI 48109, USA
E-mail address: lstruble@umich.edu

because of their comorbid medical diseases, poor health behaviors, and inadequate health care.[2,3] Health-related side effects of antipsychotic medications are also associated with increased rates of medical illness.[4] An astounding 30% to 50% of older patients who are hospitalized for a medical condition also have a psychiatric disorder.[5,6] Patients trying to adjust to multiple stressors related to an acute medical illness, new and chaotic environment, pain syndromes, aging sensory deficits, and limited coping strategies leads to an exacerbation of their psychiatric disorder and, in turn, increases the behavioral and psychiatric symptoms, length of stay, and medical complications.[7]

Typically, hospitalized older adults with psychiatric disorders have physical and cognitive impairments as well as social and financial challenges that add to the complexity in treating an acute medical illness. In addition, psychiatric disorders in older adults are also overwhelming underdiagnosed and undertreated. The hospital setting may aggravate the older person's symptoms of mental illness, and a psychiatric disorder may first be recognized in an acute medical illness situation. It is important for the astute critical care nurse to identify baseline signs and symptoms of psychiatric disorders in older patients, identify exacerbations in symptoms, seek resources, treat appropriately, and provide continuity of care during discharge planning. The intent of this article is to prepare acute care nurses to meet the mental health needs of older adults with a critical illness and prevent untoward sequelae of medical events. This article discusses the importance of baseline assessment data, addresses issues related to informed consent, and identifies successful strategies for maintaining patient safety during acute exacerbations of an acute medical illness. Common psychiatric disorders that are seen in the acute care settings are described, and strategies to improve patient outcomes are discussed.

GOALS OF CARE

Critical care nurses need to be aware of psychiatric symptoms because somatic complaints may be mistakenly attributed to a medical illness instead of the psychiatric disorder, leading to more aggressive care than may be indicated. In addition, clinicians need to recognize exacerbation of psychiatric symptoms to prevent escalations in behaviors that will make it difficult for patients to adhere to medical procedures and treatments.

Goals of care for older adults with mental illness in the acute care setting include the following:

1. Routinely assess for undiagnosed psychiatric illness in all older adults and exacerbations of psychiatric symptoms for those with an established diagnoses.
2. Recognize the special needs and unique presentation of psychiatric disorders.
3. Create an environment of safety.
4. Maintain functional abilities and strength.
5. Prevent excess disability.
6. Improve quality of life.
7. Provide continuity of care and use outpatient mental health services.

THE STIGMA OF PSYCHIATRIC DISORDERS

Psychiatric stereotypes and stigma are prevalent in today's society. Health care professionals may form strong opinions and emotional reactions to a patient's psychiatric disorder diagnosis, and his or her physical appearance or unusual behaviors may get in the way of appropriate care. Stereotypes that critical care nurses should be aware of include the following: (1) People with mental illness are always dangerous and should be avoided. (2) People with mental illness are to blame for the disabilities that arise from weak character. (3) People with mental illness are incompetent and require authority figures to make decisions for them.[8] From the classic work of Goffman,[9] the term *stigma* refers to an attribute that discredits the individual. The stigma attached to a psychiatric diagnosis causes patients to be reluctant to discuss their psychiatric history, and they attribute their current symptoms to medical conditions because it is more socially acceptable.[10] When taking care of an older adult with a psychiatric disorder, the critical care nurse needs to establish a trusting relationship and put aside old false stereotypes. Excellent communication skills are fundamentally important to elicit the patients' mood, thoughts, beliefs, and concerns. Listen to patients and empower active involvement in the decision-making process regarding their health management. Sensitive and collaborative communication is central if psychological problems are to be identified and managed.

HOSPITALIZED OLDER ADULTS

The Institute of Medicine[11] recognized the growing impact of geriatrics on health care by declaring that all providers should be competent in the care of older adults. Nowhere is this more essential than in the critical care setting where the largest cohort of patients are geriatric men and women with multiple comorbid chronic health conditions, thus creating unique challenges for care teams. Astute clinical providers and nurses should not only consider expected physiologic changes of aging adults but must also be sensitive to anxiety, delirium, substance abuse, late-onset psychiatric disorders, and unrecognized psychiatric disorders in this at-risk population.[12] Some research indicates that symptoms of depression may even instigate significant cardiac events, such as myocardial ischemia or cardiac arrest.[13] Even in healthy patients without comorbid psychiatric conditions, critical care environments are known to cause anxiety and depression that can impact patients for months after discharge from the hospital.[14] Further, Cuthbertson and colleagues[15] conducted a prospective cohort study in patients 3 months after discharge from a general critical care unit and found that 14% met the full criteria for posttraumatic stress disorder (PTSD). Other research demonstrates PTSD rates ranging from 18% to 41%,[16,17] thus significantly impacting the overall quality of life in this population of old and very old adults.

PREPARING FOR HOSPITALIZATIONS WITH PREOPERATIVE GERIATRIC ASSESSMENTS

In order to effectively intervene with critically ill elderly medical patients with comorbid psychiatric disorders, prehospitalization planning is essential. Although some admissions arrive via the emergency department, many patients are scheduled for surgical procedures in advance. In addition, some psychiatric disorders emerge in the context of a critical care hospitalization, but many are preexisting and well known to the patients, family, primary care physician, and psychiatrist. Accordingly, before admission, communication about the current psychiatric status between the psychiatric specialists and medical specialist is necessary.

The goal of the prehospitalization phase is to gather as much information as possible. This information includes the patients' current medications; allergies; results of prior psychotropic drug trials; history of medical, surgical, and psychiatric hospitalizations (suicidal/homicidal history); comorbidities; history of trauma; past and current drug use; social and occupational functioning (history of ability to relate through meaningful attachments and hold a job); adjustment to retirement; number of deaths of close people since becoming 65 years of age; as well as significant losses before becoming 65 years of age, including divorce, deaths, jobs, status. Importantly, the identification of a recent cohabiter or family member (someone who knows about recent life events and ways of living) is essential to establish a realistic baseline or to identify a history of psychiatric decompensation. Additionally, information about mental status and events leading up to the decision for hospitalization provide a useful context. Finally, names and contact information regarding current psychiatric and medical providers, legal next of kin, health care proxy, legal guardianship, as well as status of legal mental competency facilitate appropriate communication and save time. If patients were admitted emergently, a statement regarding observations before admission is useful, such as whether the patients needed to be physically or chemically restrained and the patients' response to it. Assessment of the patients' history of medication treatment adherence and the family's beliefs about the patients' illness and treatment can be instrumental in fostering an alliance with a potential support system and a partner in discharge planning.

The American College of Surgeons and the American Geriatrics Society[18] recently developed guidelines that highlight important preoperative assessments that are recommended for every geriatric surgical patient. The guidelines are comprehensive and also reflect the needs of older adults with psychiatric disorders. The preoperative assessments include cognitive impairment and dementia, decision-making ability, postoperative delirium, alcohol and substance abuse, cardiac assessment, pulmonary assessment, functional status, mobility, risk assessment for falls, frailty, nutritional status, medication regimen, counseling, preoperative testing, and patient-family and social support systems.[18]

INFORMED CONSENT ISSUES

Managing stable and unstable psychiatric conditions in an elderly population in the intensive care setting is especially challenging given the unique vulnerabilities of each of these factors (psychiatric illness, geriatric age, and complex medical care) that add complexity to the typical clinical intensive care picture of aggressive but temporary supportive medical care. Patients receiving care in the intensive care unit (ICU) often require invasive procedures for diagnostic or therapeutic purposes and may not be capable of participating in the informed consent process,[19] especially with the additional complications of psychiatric illness and cognitive changes often seen in the elderly. Clinicians need to be able to identify the essential factors that influence the ability of these vulnerable patients' ability to provide consent for treatment.

Informed consent should be viewed as a process, rather than just the signing of a document, that ensures the patients' understanding of their medical situation, serves to share pertinent medical facts and alternate courses of action, ensures the patients' capacity to understand the decision they are being asked to make, is without coercion, and includes the patients' ability to consent.[20] Among all of the factors that impact informed consent, questions of capacity and competence, defined as the ability to understand and consider medical information and then make decisions, are among the most challenging issues for providers working with acutely ill elderly patients who also have comorbid psychiatric disorders, such as depression, anxiety, PTSD, and schizophrenia. Poor energy, ambivalence, and negative thoughts that often accompany protracted critical care stays are noted in depression and physical disorders of chronic illness.[21] Further, Roberts[21] comments that other diagnoses may impede consent acquisition, such as patients with psychotic disorders who can display apathy, impaired insight, and social disengagement, whereas patients with dementia may have impaired memory and the inability to perform practical activities or even patients with substance abuse disorders because they display reduced motivation, apathy, preoccupation with substance procurement, and impaired judgment. Structured assessment tools, such as the Mini-Mental State Examination (MMSE)[22] and the MacArthur Competence Assessment Tool for Treatment[23] are objective measurements that guide the provider's decisions regarding a patient's competence.[2,24] The Montreal Cognitive Assessment (MoCA)[25] is another screening instrument that is more sensitive to picking up mild cognitive deficits and executive functioning impairments.[26]

It is essential to know that capacity of any patient may fluctuate throughout their medical course.[20] Because of this, when patients are found to be incompetent, treatment decisions should be deferred until at least 2 evaluations have been performed at another time.[27] Further, if patients are deemed to be incompetent, providers should attempt to identify and remedy the cause of the impairment before proceeding with a surrogate decision maker's consent unless the patients' medical condition warrants immediate action. In complex situations, psychiatric consultation may be warranted so that formal cognitive testing can be performed.[20,27] It is important to remember that providers are not required to obtain informed consent in emergency situations if delay of medical intervention will increase the risk of significant harm to patients and if there is a reasonable thought that the intervention will help the patients.[20] Critical care nurses and other health professionals should seek legal advice if there is any doubt regarding the legal validity of a proposed treatment.

MOOD DISORDERS

Depression and related disorders are the most common psychiatric diseases seen in older adults but often go undetected and undertreated. The prevalence of hospitalized older adults with depression ranged from 7.9% to 44.5%.[28] Somatic complaints are more common in older adults than feelings of a depressed mood. Depression is associated with many medical illnesses; if left untreated, patients can have amplified pain, delays in recovery from medical illness or surgery, increased drug side effects, cognitive decline, poor nutrition, and increased risk of suicide.[29] Older adults with the following disease states are significantly associated with depression: heart disease, stroke, Parkinson disease, dementia, and thyroid disorders. It has been reported that approximately 60% of patients who had a stroke and 45% of patients who had myocardial infarctions have depression.[30] Although there is specific diagnostic criteria to diagnose depression severity and subtypes,[31] critical care nurses need to know that any symptoms that impair physical functioning (activities of daily living), hinder the recovery or rehabilitation, or impair cognition needs to be evaluated by the psychiatry team.[32] Nurses in the acute care setting can identify or screen for possible depression and refer patients for appropriate evaluations and treatment (**Table 1**). Further, indicators that have been successful in detecting depression in hospitalized older adults include (1) recognition by treatment (eg, patients are on an antidepressant); (2) documentation by clinicians in the chart noting the following diagnosis: major depression, minor depression, dysthymic disorder, or adjustment disorder; (3) recognition of symptoms documented in the chart, such as depressed mood, sad, crying, down low, miserable, or tearful; and (4) recognition by referral, that is, recommendation for psychiatric consultation made in the chart by the physician.[33]

The prognosis for recovery with medication and psychotherapy in older adults is equal to that of younger patients. The recommended first-line treatment is the use of selective serotonin reuptake inhibitors (SSRIs) followed by tricyclic antidepressants. It should be noted that any medication for depression takes 2 to 6 weeks to achieve a therapeutic

Table 1
Common psychiatric disorders in older adults

Categories	Anxiety	Mood	Dementia	Schizophrenia	Substance Abuse
Examples of diagnosis	Generalized anxiety (GAD) Panic disorder Phobias, agoraphobia Obsessive compulsive disorder PTSD Acute stress disorder	Major depression Minor depression Bipolar disorder Psychotic depression Dysthymic disorder Adjustment disorder	Alzheimer disease Vascular dementia Parkinson disease Lewy body dementia Frontotemporal dementia	Early onset Late onset Very late onset Schizophrenialike psychosis	Substance use disorders related to the following: alcohol, amphetamines, caffeine, cannabis, cocaine, hallucinogens, inhalants, nicotine, opioids, PCP, sedative, hypnotic, or anxiolytic use Substance-induced disorders related to the following: intoxication, withdrawal, delirium, persisting dementia, persisting amnestic, psychotic, mood, anxiety, sexual dysfunction, and substance-induced sleep disorders

Symptoms				
Excessive anxiety panic	Somatic complaints	Alzheimer disease: gradual onset, mood disturbance early, psychosis and behavioral disturbances in the middle and late stages	Emotional blunting, social withdrawal, eccentric behavior, illogical thinking	Alcohol intoxication: slurred speech, incoordination, nystagmus, unsteady gait, impairment in attention or memory, stupor, or coma
Intense fear with heart pounding, nausea or GI distress, numbness, sweating, chest pain, choking feeling, fear of losing control, shaking, chills, dizziness, unsteady gait	Vague responses (eg, "I don't know" answers)	Vascular dementia: sudden onset, fluctuating course with temporary improvements and plateaus, cardiovascular disease is present and focal neurologic examination	Delusions and hallucinations less common	Alcohol withdrawal: symptoms develop within 6–8 h after last drink
Recurrent obsessions, intrusive, thoughts images, impulses causing anxiety	Reduced energy & concentration	Lewy body dementia: sudden onset; fluctuating level of awareness; psychosis, visual hallucination more prominent than delusions; parkinsonian signs, and falls	Impairment in visual-spatial tasks, mild cognitive decline over decades and is different than Alzheimer disease	Autonomic hyperactivity, mild temperature elevation (sweating, >100 pulse), Increased hand tremor, insomnia, nausea or vomiting, transient visual, tactile, or auditory hallucinations or sensory illusions, psychomotor agitation, anxiety, grand mal seizures, irritability, confusion, shaking
Compulsions, repetitive, driven behaviors to complete caused by obsession	Decreased appetite and weight loss	Frontotemporal dementias: personality changes, impaired executive function and judgment, disinhibition and social indifference; aphasia, apraxia, amnesia, and loss of calculation less prominent	Depression is common	
Behaviors excessive and aimed to reduce distress	Lack of effort while in hospital/or rehabilitation			
Intense fear related to trauma	Low self-esteem			
Recurrent intrusive thoughts or dreams of the trauma	Feelings of worthlessness			
Detached feelings	Excessive guilt			
Numbness	Sleep problems: early morning awakenings, multiple awakenings, hypersomnia			
Restricted affect	Persistent sadness, anxiety & irritability			
Increased arousal	Psychomotor agitation or retardation			
Hypervigilance, reliving the trauma	Fatigue or loss of energy[29]			
Physiologic reactivity[29]				

(continued on next page)

Table 1
(continued)

Categories	Anxiety	Mood	Dementia	Schizophrenia	Substance Abuse
Screening questions & assessment tools	Geriatric Anxiety Inventory (20 Y/N items)[82] GAD 7 screening symptoms GADSS, 6 items, older adults[83] Rating Anxiety in Dementia Scale, 20 items, cognitive impairment[84] Hospital Anxiety and Depression Scale, late life, 7 items[85]	Geriatric Depression Scale (short version), 5 items[86]	MMSE-30 items, scores <24 suggests a cognitive impairment[22] MOCA-30 items, scores <26 suggests a cognitive impairment[25] Mini Cog-5 items, a score of 0 suggests a cognitive impairment[87] CDT: patients draw a clock (do not rely on language and are nonthreatening) Score of 0 suggests a cognitive impairment[88]	Limited assessment tools Ask about symptoms, such as "Do you feel safe?"	IMADUS 20 Y/N items: 3+ positive responses indicate further assessment; questions are constructed to decrease stigma[75] CAGE 4 items: 2+ positive indicates more assessment 1+ positive response in more than 60 y suggests further asses[89] MAST-G (MI Alcohol Screening Test-Geriatric) Adaptation of MAST; 24 Y/N items: 5+ positive responses indicates further assess for use or dependence; shortened 10 items with 2+ positive response indicates ETOH problem[90]

Abbreviations: CAGE questionnaire, cut down, annoyed, guilty, and annoyed; CDT, clock drawing test; ETOH, ethyl alcohol; GAD, generalized anxiety disorder; GADSS, GAD Severity Scale; GI, gastrointestinal; IMADUS, Impressions of Medication, Alcohol, and Drug Use; MAST, Michigan Alcoholism Screening Test; MI, Michigan; mini cog, mini cognitive; PCP, phencyclidine hydrochloride; Y/N, yes/no.

response. Patients who were on an antidepressant at home should be certain to receive the medication as soon as possible if able to take it orally. If the health provider decides to start an antidepressant, make sure it is a low dose because of decreases in renal clearance and decreased ability to metabolize the drug. Additionally, in order to prevent exacerbation of bipolar disorder by using antidepressants for seemingly unipolar patients with a previously unknown or undiagnosed history of bipolar disorder, a psychiatry consult should always be considered before prescribing antidepressants.

There is a lack of scientific knowledge about bipolar disorders in older adults, and there are great variations in the presentation and course. The onset of bipolar disorders is greater in the younger population compared with older adults. Bipolar disorders have core brain features in the areas of mood, energy, cognition, and personality.[34] Bipolar I is characterized by the occurrence of one or more episodes of mania (abnormally and persistent elevated, expansive, or irritable mood) with or without an episode of depression, and bipolar II is characterized by periods of depression without episodes of mania.[35] In older adults with a bipolar disorder, there tends to be a decrease in the intensity of the extremes between depression and mania, with more frequent episodes of depression.[36] Another distinguishing factor is that there are cognitive impairments in older adults with bipolar, and late-onset bipolar is associated with more severe cognitive difficulties.[37] Older adults with depressive disorders are treated with antidepressants and antipsychotic medication. Psychotic symptoms seen in a manic episode require mood-stabilizing agents, such as lithium carbonate, lamotrigine, or divalproex, with possibly an antipsychotic medication.[38]

The act of suicide is the highest among older adults than in any other age group, especially for patients older than 85 years who are male and Caucasian. The characteristics of suicide in older adults include the following: Patients use more lethal methods with higher percentages of completed suicides.[39] Patients are less likely to have discussed their plans beforehand.[40] Nonviolent deaths from suicide may be mistakenly attributed to illness.[39] Comorbid depression and disruption and/or a lack of social support is significantly associated with suicide in late life.[41] In one study,[42] the following specific illnesses were associated with suicide in older adults: congestive heart failure, chronic obstructive lung disease, seizure disorder, urinary incontinence, anxiety disorders, psychotic disorders, bipolar disorder, and moderate to severe pain. The risk was also greatly increased when the patients had multiple illnesses. Acute care nurses can impact suicide mortality. The assessment should focus on the patients' immediate suicide risks, identifying increased or severe psychiatric symptoms, and determining if older patients who refuse treatments or are trying to leave the hospital are mentally fit to decline help. Whenever possible, obtain collateral information from family members regarding the patients' behaviors (eg, stock piling pills, recent purchase of a gun, or giving away personal belongings) to help determine the risk of suicide. For more information, see Holkup[43] for a nurse protocol that provides assessments on suicidality in older adults.

ANXIETY

Anxiety symptoms and disorders rank among the most common psychiatric problems in people of all ages and affect large numbers of older adults.[44] Following the Surgeon General's 1999 Mental Health Report,[45] which emphasized the importance of identifying and treating psychiatric disorders and mental distress in older adults, hundreds of studies of depression, pain, and dementia emerged.[46] Studies of anxiety in older adults, on the other hand, were comparatively few. Although symptoms of anxiety in older adults are commonly present in primary care (14.5%–19.5%), anxiety disorders are notably less recognized, undertreated, or otherwise diagnosed as evidenced in the older adult research literature.[47,48] In the ICU, for example, the exact prevalence of older adult anxiety disorders still remains unclear, but their presence is palpable. Sources of ICU anxiety in the older adult range from difficulty communicating, fear, and worrying about location of hearing aids and glasses, to premorbid psychiatric illnesses and personality disorders. Indeed, the very nature of anxiety symptom presentations (eg, vague descriptions, worry, emotionality, cognitive blocking, memory interference, apprehension, somatic symptoms, agitation, apprehension, restlessness, irritation) are sometimes experienced by professionals as frustrating annoyances versus representations of anxiety symptom clusters. Because many older people do not seek psychiatric treatment, the private use of alternative sources of comfort (eg, alcohol, sedatives, and so forth) leads to serious clinical problems when critical care is necessary. These problems include withdrawal syndromes and increased anxiety with admission to the acute care environment. Failure to appropriately identify anxiety disorders in older adults leads to misdiagnosis; unrecognized problems; inappropriate treatment; and, most importantly, missed opportunities to treat treatable problems.

Early assessment through screening for anxiety disorders is essential in the acute care of older adult patients because of the patients' capacity to deteriorate quickly. Anxiety screening tools, such as the Generalized Anxiety Scale, the Rating Anxiety in Dementia Scale, and the Hospital Anxiety and Depression Scale are short, efficient screening aids that facilitate the identification of symptoms in the acute care setting. Specific symptom identification optimizes the likelihood of accurate treatment recommendations when making a psychiatry referral. Accurate critical nursing assessment of anxiety in older adults also requires an appreciation of 2 factors: first, a variety of neurologic, endocrine, respiratory, cardiovascular, and metabolic illnesses may be causing the anxiety; second, the subcategories of anxiety diagnoses that are subsumed under the general area of anxiety disorder–related problems are unique relative to each other in their origins, causes, and presentations. These categories (**Table 2**) include generalized anxiety disorder, anxiety disorder caused by a medical disorder, substance use, agoraphobia, panic disorder (with and without agoraphobia), social phobia, specific phobias, obsessive-compulsive disorder, and PTSD. Astute critical care nursing observation of the emergence, timing, and manifestation of anxiety symptoms is extremely useful in planning appropriate intervention. The utilization of prehospitalization psychiatric history information or the implementation of an anxiety screening tool could allow the development of an intervention plan for the emergence of anxiety-related problems. For example, an older woman's terrified screams in the ICU when being undressed for bathing could be potentially averted by the knowledge that she has a diagnosis of PTSD exacerbated by being touched by strangers. For her, PTSD symptoms include periodic flashbacks and lashing out comparable with how one might behave when attacked in a violent gang rape. If well-meaning attempts to contain her anxiety or protect her from pulling out her tubing are dealt with by the use of quickly imposed physical restraint, further delay of necessary medical treatment might occur. Chaos and detained medical care would ensue as the patient resisted bodily restraint/confinement against her wishes. Careful screening and communication could enhance effective management and care. Likewise, in other cases, early identification of a panic disorder or phobia history could allow for accurate decision making to use preprocedure anxiety medication before magnetic resonance imaging in phobic patients. A brief assessment could have led to individualized planning versus patient embarrassment, extra staff time, and increased institutional cost for the delayed procedure.

Table 2
Nonpharmacological interventions for older adults with psychiatric disorders

Geriatric, Mental Health, and Hospital Issues	Interventions
Hearing changes	• Support the use of patients' hearing aids or provide other hearing amplifiers (electronic or use your stethoscope and speak softly into bell) • Keep face visible and allow patients to see your lips (eg, talk to patients before you put your mask on) • Use touch to get patients' attention (monitor for startle reflex and comfort level) • Position yourself at the same level as patients • Enunciate clearly and slowly in a low-pitched voice • Use short sentence and repeat • Do not change topic abruptly • Ask clear and precise questions • Use visual cues
Hearing voices and noises	• Assess whether auditory hallucination present or misperception (eg, ventilator is steam engine or monitor is fire alarm, cannot see the person behind the curtain who is talking, perceives what is on TV) • Evaluate if voices are telling patients to harm themselves or others • Evaluate whether voices are extremely upsetting to patients and how they are coping with the voices • Order a psychiatric consult • Evaluate for antipsychotic medications
Vision changes	• Support use of patients' glasses or provide magnifying glass • Avoid glare: windows or lights • Develop appropriate visual materials: at least 12-point type font, double space with a lot of white space between chunks of information
Communication difficulties	• Allow patients time to respond to a question (time how long it takes, sometimes it can be 60–90 seconds) • Avoid negative tone or criticism • Treat patients as individuals with feelings • Do not talk over patients as if they are not there • Give clear simple written and verbal information early and often; check the patients' comprehension and recall • Avoid using jargon and detailed complex information • Encourage patients to ask questions
Difficulty establishing relationships and trust	• Establish rapport • Speak in calm, reassuring voice; no baby talk • Person-centered care • Consistent staff • Always introduce yourself and your role • Discuss what tasks you are going to perform before proceeding • Encourage family and friend contacts

(continued on next page)

Table 2
(continued)

Geriatric, Mental Health, and Hospital Issues	Interventions
Overstimulating physical environment	• Simplify environment by eliminating noise and distractions • Remove clutter
Understimulating physical environment	• Soothing music of patients' choice • Simple activities
Mobility limitations and falls	• Encourage physical activity • Walking patients if possible every shift • Bed in low position, consider mat next to bed • Anticipate needs • Bathroom schedule • Refer to physical therapy
Cognitive difficulties	• Ensure you have patients' attention • Use the patients' last name and title to refocus their attention • Divide tasks into simple steps • Eliminate distractions • Provide memory devices: clocks, calendars • Large-print written reminders of scheduled treatments, tests, and family visits • Encourage visitors to write encouraging messages in a notebook and the times that they visited • Encourage family to bring in familiar objects • Place family pictures, especially those from their younger days in a prominent place • Reinforce routines • Keep tasks within the patients' capabilities
Loss of independence caused by acute illness	• Avoid use of restraints when possible (restraints may increase agitation) • Occupational therapy referral for adaptive devices • Allow freedom of movement in a supervised, safe environment • Movement alarms
Nutrition and eating difficulties	• Encourage patients to brush teeth before meals • Ensure dentures are in place • Sit in chair for all meals • Use placemat if possible to establish the eating area with contrasting color plate • Use familiar objects that reinforce the eating experience (eg, clear plastic cup so can see what is in cup verses carton or styrofoam) • Small frequent meals • Encourage family to bring in food

Nonpharmacological treatment of anxiety disorders in older adult critical care patients is complicated by the fast pace and intense activity typical of the acute care setting. Relaxation therapy, cognitive behavioral techniques, and supportive therapy have research support for the treatment of late-life anxiety disorders according to systematic reviews and research critiques.[49–51] Yet, the state of the science is such that it is unclear whether preprocedure use of nonpharmacological interventions is the optimal intervention for anxiety reduction in the acute care arena.

Pharmacologic interventions for anxiety disorders are based primarily on their use with younger populations. However, Andrade[52] notes that the SSRIs are the first-line medications for the pharmacologic treatment of anxiety disorders in the elderly because of both the efficacy and having the most favorable side-effect profile. Specifically, citalopram, sertraline, venlafaxine, and buspirone are drugs for which there is at least modest empiric data; tiagabine, on the other hand, is an effective drug for which use is specifically discouraged.[52] It should be noted that citalopram should be maintained at a low dose (10 mg/d) and, like sertraline, has minimal P450 drug interactions; venlafaxine has the potential to increase blood pressure at higher doses (>100 mg/d); buspirone does not induce withdrawal or dependence syndromes.[53] Unfortunately, the initiation of SSRI treatment in the acute care arena will provide limited anxiety reduction at best because of the 2- to 6-week start-up time necessary for a therapeutic response. However, psychiatry consultation could facilitate the decision making regarding the initiation of SSRI use to facilitate the patients' transition to rehabilitation or home, particularly for those benzodiazepine-dependent patients who think continued benzodiazepine use is necessary. Although short-acting benzodiazepines can be used temporarily in the acute care setting for anxiety and agitation reduction because of their quick and effective response, knowledge of the patients' prior use and abuse of them is essential so as to not contribute to relapse. Lauderdale and Sheikh[54] note that continuous use of benzodiazepines for greater than 6 weeks would require a treatment plan that includes a gradual taper over the next several weeks. Because of both the sedation and dependence potential, benzodiazepine use in the acute care setting should be restricted to older adult patients who fall into 4 categories: (1) those for whom rapid anxiety reduction is required; (2) those requiring a short duration of treatment, such as patients with acute stress disorder or an adjustment disorder; (3) those who are terminally ill; and (4) those patients who have had an inadequate response to anxiolytics from other classes.

DEMENTIA

Dementia is a nonspecific illness syndrome. It is not a normal part of aging, but it is a serious, progressive neurologic and psychiatric disorder that affects 13 out of 1000 patients aged 65 to 69 years and 122 out of 1000 patients aged older than 80 years.[55] Dementia is defined as an impairment of memory and the loss of at least one of the following: language (aphasia); reasoning and planning (executive function); orientation; regulation of mood or changes in personality; and recognition and manipulation of objects (agnosia, apraxia), calculations, and attention of sufficient severity to interfere with social and occupational functioning.

Dementia is only a descriptive term and the specific type or diagnosis is important to determine to provide optimal treatment interventions. It is a terminal disease requiring palliative care interventions, but unfortunately only half of the patients with dementia have even been diagnosed.[55] Older patients with undiagnosed dementia may display significant symptoms for the first time when hospitalized with a medical illness. The symptoms will become increasingly apparent when the patients are stressed from an unfamiliar environment and medical illness. Patients with dementia are at increased risk of delirium. It is important to define, if possible, the type of dementia because there are specific distinguishing features and disease pathophysiology that determine optimal treatments.

Alzheimer disease is the most common type of dementia and accounts for approximately 80% of the cases. Other common types of dementia include vascular dementia, mixed dementia (Alzheimer and vascular), Lewy body dementia, Parkinson with dementia, and frontotemporal dementia. A very important feature to remember is that all patients with dementia are alert and awake, unlike other types of brain disorders, until the later stages when there may be fluctuations in consciousness. There is one exception: patients with Lewy body dementia commonly have transient, unexplained loss of consciousness that, in part, may be related to severe autonomic dysfunction.[56]

Identifying the stage of dementia (mild, moderate, and severe) is important so that nursing interventions related to communication, performing tasks, and maintaining the patients' functional abilities are met without causing the patients and/or nurse frustration or distress. Often, short-term memory loss is the first sign of dementia; the patients' ability to process and remember information and problem solve during a medical crises deteriorates quickly. The hospital setting is quite challenging for patients with dementia because cognitive and function abilities rapidly decline in an unfamiliar physical and social environment. In the moderate stages of dementia, cognitive abilities decrease, functional autonomy is lost, and behavioral symptoms become increasingly problematic. Any new hospital procedure may trigger anxiety and fear, and patients may strongly resist or withdraw from the perceived threats. Malnutrition and dehydration are also common because patients may not be able to recognize or communicate their needs. A hospital food tray does not look like the familiar family place setting at home. Cartons of milk or packaged hospital food may not be recognizable to the person with dementia. Monitor for swallowing difficulties and allow patients to sit in the chair for meals whenever possible. Problems with gait and abnormal movements (including bradykinesia, Parkinsonism, rigidity, multifocal myoclonus, tendency to fall, and so forth) are very prevalent in patients with dementia. Palliative care is needed throughout the disease process and does not hasten the death of patients with dementia. The focus should be on relieving symptoms, such as pain, shortness of breath, fatigue, nausea, loss of appetite, and difficulty sleeping. Hospice care should be considered in the late stages of dementia.[57]

Neuropsychiatric symptoms are extremely common, with prevalence rates estimated between 61% and 88%[58]; as dementia progresses and aphasia increases, people with dementia express their emotions nonverbally in the form of behaviors. Common behaviors that may be seen in hospitalized patients with dementia include physically aggressive (hitting, biting, scratching); physically nonaggressive behaviors (pacing, rummaging, wandering); verbal agitation (yelling, swearing, repetitive vocalizations); psychiatric symptoms (eg, delusions, hallucinations); inappropriate sexual behavior and other forms of disinhibition (spitting, rude comments); mood disturbance (eg, apathy, depression, euphoria, emotional lability); and neurovegetative changes (eg, appetite changes, sleep disturbance).[59,60] In part, the frequency, intensity, and type of behavioral symptoms vary and depend on the specific type of dementia. For example, people with Lewy body dementia experience a higher incidence of hallucinations; people with vascular dementia commonly express more depressive and emotional lability; and frontotemporal dementia is characterized by disinhibition, apathy, and social inappropriateness.[61]

The use of cholinesterase inhibitors is a palliative treatment of patients with dementia. The use of cholinesterase inhibitors, such as donepezil (Aricept), rivastigmine (Exelon), and galantamine (Razadyne), may delay cognitive decline, improve the ability to perform activities of daily living, improve cognition, and improve psychological and behavioral disturbances, including psychosis.[62] The other category of medications specifically for moderate to severe dementia is an N-methyl-D-aspartate receptor antagonist memantine (Namenda). Patients should continue these medications, if at all possible, during their hospital stay. Abrupt stopping of the medication could result in significant cognitive decline, falls, and increased neuropsychiatric behaviors. If patients have been off of the medications for several days, medications should be restarted at the lowest dose and titrated up because of the potential gastrointestinal adverse reactions (nausea, vomiting, diarrhea, loss of appetite). The use of antipsychotic medications for psychotic and aggressive behaviors is associated with higher mortality rates than other drug categories used for behavioral symptoms. The cause is not well understood and may be from the antipsychotic medication's effect or the pathophysiology underlying the neuropsychiatric symptoms.[63] Nonpharmacological interventions are the first-line treatment of behavioral disturbances.

SCHIZOPHRENIA

Schizophrenia begins in late adolescence or young adulthood, usually before 45 years of age; the disease persists throughout life. The number of patients with schizophrenia is expected to double to 1 million in the next 20 years.[64] Late-onset schizophrenia (after 40 years of age) and very-late-onset schizophrenialike psychosis (after 60 years of age) can also occur; therefore, the diagnosis of schizophrenia should not be excluded based on the age at onset.[65] The positive symptoms seen in schizophrenia include delusions (most common theme is persecutory delusions whereby patients think they are under surveillance), hallucinations (hearing voices is the most common type), thought disorders (trouble organizing their thoughts or connecting them logically), and movement disorders (most common are agitated body movements or repetition of certain motions; catatonia is rare). Negative symptoms in schizophrenia are defined as disruptions in emotions and behaviors (eg, flat affect, lack of speech, anhedonia, and inability to initiate or sustain planned activities). Cognitive symptoms are subtle and difficult to recognize but can be detected with screening assessments (eg, poor executive function, poor attention span, inability to use information immediately after learning it).[66] Hospitalized older adults with schizophrenia will need help with everyday tasks and basic personal hygiene. Published research on older adults with schizophrenia is very limited. It is estimated that only 1% of the research data on schizophrenia is specific to older adults in the past decade.[67] Although information is limited, there is an age-associated decrease in dopaminergic and other monoaminergic activities that may decrease the severity of psychotic symptoms in older adults. About 20% of patients with schizophrenia show no active symptoms by 65 years of age.[68] Sustained remission and a better prognosis with a decrease and discontinuation of antipsychotics have been observed. The factors that contribute to a better prognosis include the following: female gender, later disease onset (aged in the 40s–50s), married, and appropriate early treatment.[64] Social support is very important; if social connections are made before the illness or they have strong family-patient advocates, they use health care services and have better patient outcomes. The maintenance of psychopharmacologic agents is important in the hospital setting, and critical care nurses need to observe for extrapyramidal side effects and tardive dyskinesia. Older adults respond well to psychopharmacological agents; usually, medications should be at lower-than-usual doses. Some patients may be tapered off the medication in late adulthood.

SUBSTANCE USE

The literature on substance use shows considerable variation in reports of, attention to, and recognition of the extent of the problem of substance use disorders in older adults. Those who are particularly attuned to its prevalence, the Substance Abuse and Mental Health Services Administration [SAMHSA][69] note that in their 2007 national survey including 2426 adults older than 65 years, lifetime illicit drug use was reported in 10.7% of the sample; 39.1% indicated some alcohol use in the past month. An estimate of prevalence rates for 2020 based on 1999 SAMHSA data projected that the number of those who were alcohol or drug dependent at 50 years of age or older would increase from 500,000 to 700,000 by 2020.[69] Additionally, those who drank heavily or used illicit drugs would increase from 930,000 to 1.1 million by 2020. Accordingly, as the baby boomer generation ages (ie, those born between 1946 and 1964 who used drugs and alcohol in their adolescence and early adulthood more than any previous generation), a clear increase in legal and illegal substance use is expected in our patient population. These data suggest that substance use and the multiple comorbidities from histories of long-term substance use may profoundly influence the nature of acute care admissions in the near future.

According to Savage,[70(pp265)] the term *substance abuse* refers to "use of a substance or substances in an uncontrolled, compulsive, and potentially harmful manner." The diagnosis of substance abuse according to the American Psychiatric Association[31] requires evidence of a maladaptive pattern of substance use in a 12-month period of time resulting in an accompanying impairment in one of 4 areas of function. These areas include impairment in social and/or occupational functioning (eg, school, job, or home responsibilities), legal problems, risk of danger caused by the use of a substance (eg, driving a car while under the influence), and ongoing interpersonal problems resulting from or brought on by substance use.

Screening for substance use disorders in the older adult population, particularly in the critical care arena, is essential for several reasons. First, substance use is rarely a prominent part of the medical record; thus, a history of use is not immediately evident. Second, substance use has the potential to interfere with the action of pharmacologic agents in critical care. Third, substance use is often inaccurately reported or unrecognized as a problem by patients and/or family members. The primary screening tools available (see **Table 1**) focus on alcohol abuse, the most significant substance use disorder for older adults. Carlat[71] notes that approaching alcohol screening in a nonjudgmental way (eg, Do you have a drink now and then? versus How much do you drink?) before asking formal screening questions yields significantly greater sensitivity to responses. Eliason[72] emphasizes the importance of a full biopsychosocial assessment, noting that the diagnosis of patients with decades of substance use can be confounded by what seems to be a clinical presentation of dementia, resulting in the potential for misdiagnosis.

The current diagnostic categorization of substance related disorders in the *Diagnostic and Statistical Manual of Mental Disorders* (Fourth Edition, Text Revision)[31] is divided into 2 groups consisting of substance use disorders (ie, substance dependence and abuse) and substance-induced (SI) disorders (eg, SI intoxication, SI withdrawal, SI delirium, SI persisting dementia, and so forth). Yet the most common substance problem in the older adult population in the critical care arena is related to alcohol. Fingerhood[73] identified 2 categories of alcoholism for older adults. The first, *early onset* alcohol abuse, contains 66% of older adult alcohol abusers who tend to drink until intoxicated; have more legal, occupational, and financial problems; have less social support; and have been in unsuccessful treatment of alcoholism in the past. As a result, many have impaired cognition with chronic health problems. The second category, *late-onset* alcohol abuse, contains people whose alcohol abuse begins after 60 years of age, are more likely to be depressed or feel lonely, typically enter treatment resulting from a crisis, deny alcohol problem, and have a support system in family or friends.[73,74] The stress of aging (eg, retirement, disability, loss of sensory capabilities, financial and health problems, and reduced ability of an older body to manage alcohol) contributes to the development of late-onset alcoholism.[75] Although alcohol withdrawal syndromes are typically well handled by the expertise of the critical care team, complexities exist with the management of severe alcohol problems in the elderly. Notably, when neurologic complications of severe alcoholism interface with the cognitive changes associated with age, a confusing picture may emerge. Complications include Wernicke encephalopathy, Korsakoff psychosis, and alcoholic dementia. Wernicke encephalopathy is characterized by an acute confusional state, lateral gaze abnormalities, ataxia, and nystagmus. It is caused by thiamin deficiency and reversed by treatment with thiamin replacement followed by glucose administration.[76] Korsakoff psychosis can result from untreated encephalopathy, presents with amnesia and confabulation, has permanent memory impairment, does not respond to thiamin replacement, has an unknown cause, and is irreversible.[77,78] Alcohol-induced dementia resembles Alzheimer disease, but frontal lobe symptoms (eg, apathy) along with intellectual and other cognitive losses caused by alcoholic brain damage leave patients unresponsive to typical Alzheimer treatments.

The management of the substance use disorders in the critical care arena provides nursing staff with a unique opportunity to facilitate a life-altering change. Serious attention to the importance of follow-up should be an integral part of the treatment plan such that an identified care manager follows through with patients after discharge until the connection is made with Alcoholics Anonymous, Narcotics Anonymous, or the appropriate local substance use treatment facility. Resistance should be anticipated; but denial will not change without the committed, but sensitive effort at breaking through the resistance. Research by Atkinson[79] and Blow[80] show that older adult men and women respond better to substance abuse treatment programs that are designed for their age, include individual counseling, have a slower pace, attend to comorbid psychiatric and medical problems, and use nonconfrontational approaches to treatment.

BEHAVIORAL APPROACHES FOR OLDER ADULTS WITH PSYCHIATRIC DISORDERS

Health care professionals and family caregivers alike want to control behaviors and have older patients with mental health issues act normal, which is not possible. Understanding that neuropsychiatric behaviors are part of a brain disease will help nurses develop behavioral strategies and be more tolerant of annoying behaviors that do not risk the safety of either the patients or health care professionals. Behavioral symptoms are a way of communicating needs, such as distress, fear, and pain. Recognizing older patients' emotional and cognitive abilities will help nurses to develop interventions that will improve the patients' level of functioning and comfort. Documenting the behavior in terms of specific descriptions of the antecedent to the behaviors (morning dressing change), what the behavior was in detail (patient started screaming and hit the nurse in the patient's room at 3 PM when dressing change started), and the consequences of the behavior (patient very upset and dressing did not get changed, nurse was injured) will help in determining the cause of the disruptive behavior and in developing interventions. Assess and document the following: body language and voice; hyposensitivity or hypersensitivity to stimulation for vision, hearing, touch, taste and smell; the behavior; level of functioning; and strengths and coping styles. See **Table 2** for possible interventions.

CASE

A common case typically seen in a critical care setting is presented. Given your understanding of psychiatric conditions, how would you provide care to a 72-year-old man with a history of type 2 diabetes mellitus, gout, PTSD, and depression who was just admitted to the cardiovascular intensive care unit for hypertension management and evaluation of a thoracic aortic aneurysm? The patient, a retired welder, was divorced 33 years ago and currently lives alone. He is estranged from his 2 sons who live out of state. The patient reports a 40 pack-year tobacco history and drinks 4 to 6 beers per day most days. Preoperatively, he was started on folic acid, thiamine, multivitamin, and lorazepam. The patient had a successful surgical repair of his aortic valve and thoracic aortic aneurysm; but postoperatively, he was very agitated, required several days of intravenous esmolol to control his hypertension, and was not able to be extubated until the fourth postoperative day. On postoperative day 8, the patient became febrile and hypotensive. The patient was started on broad-spectrum antibiotics and required volume resuscitation, pressor support, and eventually intermittent dialysis because of the development of acute kidney injury. Over the last few days, the patient has become more withdrawn, is having trouble sleeping, and does not want to participate in his physical therapy program. He tells the nurse that he is too tired to go on. The medical team has been unable to make contact with any of his family despite several attempts.

Positive blood cultures and a new diastolic murmur prompted transesophageal echocardiography, which revealed an aortic root abscess. The surgeon and critical care team determine that the patient will require an immediate redo aortic valve and aortic root repair to resolve his infection. The surgeon is anxious to get the patient to surgery. After speaking with the patient, the surgeon asks the nurse practitioner to prepare the patient's preoperative orders and obtain consent; however, she is concerned that the patient may not be able to give consent because of his confounding complex medical course complicated by his deepening depressive symptoms. What strategies should the team use to minimize the impact of the patient's past medical history of PTSD, substance use, and depression in the midst of his complex medical situation? How would you manage this situation with his consent?

CARE FOR PATIENTS: CASE EXAMPLE

In providing care to the aforementioned case, the impact of the patient's past medical history of PTSD, substance use, and depression on his current hospitalization is significant and unfortunate. Preoperative planning using facts that should be preoperatively available to the team (assuming electronic record and permission/access to view other records) would include knowledge that the patient has 3 chronic medical illnesses (diabetes, gout, and hypertension) that require self-management skills for healthy living. A psychiatric assessment (or even a psychiatric review of the record) would have predicted a pattern of psychological and physical dependence (in his 40 pack-year cigarette and 4–6 daily beer habit, likely a minimal estimate) suggesting a limited ability to address self-care needs and significantly challenged self-comfort/self-soothing abilities. With this assessment, one would assume that withdrawal from maladaptive coping efforts (smoking and drinking) would leave him at even greater risk for increased anxiety, depression, irritability, and agitation when confronted with physical withdrawal from his usual friends (ie, tobacco and beer). His profoundly deplete lack of social support (retired, divorced, lives alone, estranged from 2 sons) limits other options and complicates matters when the team needs to make on-the-spot management decisions with minimal cooperation from a patient whose judgment is chemically compromised. A psychiatry consult as early as possible during the patient's hospitalization is essential for this man in light of his worsening depression (increased withdrawal, sleep disturbance, decreased motivation, and possible suicidal ideation) after developing complications from the first surgery.

Psychiatry would be in a better position to assess and work with the team regarding the following:

1. Obtain the previous psychiatric and family psychiatric history, including previous diagnoses, severity of symptoms, as well as previous suicidality, psychiatric hospitalizations, and psychiatric medication trials. These data would be used in formulating an appropriate psychiatric diagnosis, medication, and treatment plan.
2. Assess for Suicidality (ie, active thoughts, intent, plan, previous attempts, ability to let staff know of worsening thoughts, and so forth).
3. PTSD: Develop an understanding of the nature and impact of the original trauma, whether this man is still having symptoms and, if so, how serious they are or whether the symptoms are primarily residual and not currently impacting his life. Further, has the man developed any new symptoms related to whether the surgery and the complicated medical course during this hospitalization might have been traumatic? If symptoms of PTSD (flashbacks of trauma, avoidance of trauma reminders, nightmares, and so forth) are not interfering with his present care, this could be evaluated further as an outpatient and evaluated for whether treatment is needed. An antidepressant (SSRI) might be helpful if he is having active symptoms, particularly if they persist on an outpatient basis.
4. Substance use: The administration of the Michigan Alcohol Withdrawal Severity assessment scale could occur by either a general physician or a psychiatry specialist, followed by a detoxification protocol based on the assessment results. It is a good decision to use lorazepam. An outpatient extended evaluation and treatment would be important discharge recommendations.

Useful registered nurse interventions might include the following:

1. Set aside 10 to 15 minutes of uninterrupted time each shift to connect with the patients to decrease isolation and offer comfort and support.
2. Explore ways for the patient to receive emotional comfort. Assess adaptive possibilities (vs smoking and drinking) for self-soothing and comfort during difficult times.
3. Assess whether the patient might like to speak to a member of the clergy or hospital social worker.
4. Evaluate whether there are friends he would like to speak to or visit with.
5. Encourage the patient to express his feelings about his situation or write them in a journal.
6. Offer pleasant distraction activities, including television, games, reading, music, time with staff, and so forth.
7. Assess the patient's mood and risk for suicide each shift, and increase the frequency of monitoring for suicidality as appropriate.
8. Monitor for possible medication side effects of SSRI (nausea, drowsiness, headache, activation, and so forth).

SUMMARY

Complications from psychiatric disorders along with medical disorders treated in critical care are often reciprocally complicating. Psychiatric patients' stability may be challenged by the speed, chaos, and physical intrusions imposed by medical treatments in a medical emergency department or ICU; likewise, newly stabilized medical/surgical ICU patients may become quickly destabilized by the psychiatric patients' paranoid delusions brought on by unanticipated medication interactions. Treatment of each is complex; treatment of both simultaneously is an art.

Prehospitalization preparation, family communication, team collaboration, and a calm focus on the patients' mental status are essential to minimizing additional stress for all involved. In fact, the patients' treatment can be seriously compromised after discharge if the families do not consider themselves allies in the treatment.[81]

REFERENCES

1. Jeste DV, Alexopoulos GS, Bartels SJ, et al. Consensus statement on the up-coming crisis in geriatric mental health: research agenda for the next 2 de-cades. Arch Gen Psychiatry 1999;56:848–53.
2. Baxter DN. The mortality experience of individuals on the Salford Psychiatric Case Register. Br J Psychiatry 1996;168:772–9.
3. Jeste DV, Gladsjo JA, Lindamer LA, et al. Medical comorbidity in schizophrenia. Schizophr Bull 1996;22:413–30.
4. DeHert M, Dekker JM, Wood D, et al. Cardiovascular disease and diabetes in people with severe mental illness position statement from the European Psychiatric Association (EPA), supported by the European Association for the Study of Diabetes (EASD) and the European Society of Cardiology (ESC). Eur Psychiatry 2009;24:412–24.
5. Rapp SR, Parisi SA, Walsh DA. Psychological dysfunction and physical health among elderly medical inpatients. J Consult Clin Psychol 1988;56:851–5.
6. Spar JE, La Rue A. An aging world. In: Spar JE, LaRue A, editors. A clinical manual of geriatric psychiatry. Arlington (TX): VA American Psychiatric Publishing Inc; 2006. p. 6–15.
7. Unutzer J, Patrick DL, Simon G, et al. Depressive symptoms and the cost of health services in HMO patients aged 65 years and older. J Am Med Assoc 1997;277:1618–23.
8. Corrigan PW, Green A, Lundin R, et al. Familiarity with and social distance from people who have serious mental illness. Psychiatr Serv 2001;52:553–8.
9. Goffman E. Stigma: notes on the management of spoiled identity. Englewood Cliffs (NJ): Prentice-Hall; 1963.
10. Staab JP, Datto CJ, Weinrieb RB, et al. Detection and diagnosis of psychiatric disorders in primary medical care settings. Med Clin North Am 2001;85:579–96.
11. Institute of Medicine. Retooling for an aging America. Building the healthcare workforce. Washington, DC: National Academy Press; 2008.
12. Patusky KL, Caldwell B, Unkle D, et al. Incorporating the treatment of medical and psychiatric disorders in the critical care area. Crit Care Nurs Clin North Am 2012;24:53–80.
13. Grewal K, Stewart DE, Abbey SE, et al. Timing of depressive symptom onset and in-hospital complications among acute coronary syndrome in patients. Psychosomatics 2010;51:283–8.
14. Jones C, Skirrow P, Griffiths RD, et al. Rehabilitation after critical illness: a randomized, controlled trial. Crit Care Med 2003;31:2458–61.
15. Cuthbertson BH, Hull A, Stracham M, et al. Post-traumatic stress disorder after critical illness requiring general intensive care. Intensive Care Med 2004;30:450–5.
16. Scragg P, Jones A, Fauvel N. Psychological problems following ICU treatment. Anesthesia 2001;56:9–14.
17. Stoll C, Schelling G, Goetz A, et al. Health-related quality of life and post-traumatic stress disorder in patients after cardiac surgery and intensive care treatment. J Thorac Cardiovasc Surg 2000;120:505–12.

18. Chow WB, Rosenthal RA, Merkow RP, et al. Optimal preoperative assessment of the geriatric surgical patient: a best practices guideline from the American College of Surgeons National Surgical Quality Improvement Program and the American Geriatrics Society. J Am Coll Surg 2012;215:453–66.
19. Davis N, Pohlman A, Gehlbach B, et al. Improving the process of informed consent in the critically ill. J Am Med Assoc 2003;289:1963–8.
20. Terry PB. Informed consent in clinical medicine. Chest 2007;131(2):563–8.
21. Roberts LW. Informed consent and the capacity for voluntarism. Am J Psychiatry 2002;159:705–12.
22. Folstein MF, Folstein SE, McHugh PR. "Mind-mental state": a practical method for grading the cognitive state of patients for the clinician. J Psychiatr Res 1975;12:189–98.
23. Grisso T, Appelbaum PS. Macarthur Competence Assessment Tool for Treatment (MacCAT-T). Sarasota (FL): Professional Resource Press; 1998.
24. Raymont V, Bingley W, Buchanan A, et al. Prevalence of mental incapacity in medical inpatients and associated risk factors: cross sectional study. Lancet 2004;364:1421–7.
25. Nasreddine ZS, Phillips NA, Bedirian V, et al. The Montreal Cognitive Assessment (MoCA): a brief screening tool for mild cognitive impairment. J Am Geriatr Soc 2005;53(4):695–9.
26. Dong Y, Sharma VK, Chan BP, et al. The Montreal Cognitive Assessment (MoCA) is superior to the Mini-Mental State Examination (MMSE) for the detection of vascular cognitive impairment after acute stroke. J Neurol Sci 2010;299:15–8.
27. Appelbaum PS. Assessment of patients' competence to consent to treatment. N Engl J Med 2007;357:1834–40.
28. McCusker J, Cole M, Ciampi A, et al. Twelve-month trajectories of depressive symptoms in older medical inpatients. Am J Geriatr Psychiatry 2007;22:411–7.
29. Harvath TA, McKenzie G. Depression in older adults. In: Boltz M, Capezuti E, Fulmer T, et al, editors. Evidence-based geriatric nursing protocols for best practice. 4th edition. New York (NY): Springer Publishing Company; 2012. p. 135–62.
30. Raj A. Depression in the elderly: tailoring medical therapy to their needs. Postgrad Med 2004;115:26–42.
31. American Psychiatric Association. Diagnostic and statistical manual of mental disorder: DSM-IV-TR. Text revision. 4th edition. Washington, DC: Author; 2000.
32. Koenig HG, Blazer DG. Mood disorders. In: Blazer DG, Steffens DC, Busse EW, editors. Textbook of geriatric psychiatry. Arlington (VA): American Psychiatric Publishing, Inc; 2004. p. 241.
33. Cepoiu M, McCusker J, Cole M, et al. Recognition of depression in older medical inpatients. J Gen Intern Med 2007;22:559–63.
34. Depp CA, Jeste DV. Bipolar disorder in older adults: a critical review. Bipolar Disord 2004;6:343–67.
35. Beers MH, Berkow R. Merck manual of geriatrics. 3rd edition. Whitehouse Station (NJ): Merck Research Laboratories; 2000.
36. National Institutes of Mental Health. A story of bipolar disorder. 2002. Available at: www.nimh, nih.gov/pub licat/bipolarstory08.cfm. Accessed November 16, 2012.
37. Schouws S, Comijs HC, Tek ML, et al. Cognitive impairment in early and late bipolar disorder. Am J Geriatr Psychiatry 2009;17:508–14.
38. Zayas EM, Grossberg GT. The treatment of psychosis in late life. J of Clinical Psychiatry 1998;59(Suppl 1):5–10.
39. Cornwell Y. Suicide among elderly persons. Psychiatr Serv 1995;46:563–4.

40. Carney SS, Rich CL, Burke PA, et al. Suicide over 60: the San Diego study. J Am Geriatr Soc 1994;42:174–80.
41. Conwell Y, Duberstein PR, Caine ED. Risk factors for suicide in later life. Biol Psychiatry 2002;52:193–204.
42. Juurlink DN, Herrmann N, Szalai J, et al. Medical illness and the risk of suicide in the elderly. Arch Intern Med 2004;164:1179–84.
43. Holkup PA. Evidence based protocol: elderly suicide secondary prevention. J Gerontol Nurs 2003;29:6–17.
44. Kessler RC, Berglund P, Demler O, et al. Lifetime prevalence and age-of-onset distributions of DSM-IV disorders in the National Co-Morbidity Survey replication. Arch Gen Psychiatry 2005;62:593–602.
45. U.S. Department of Health and Human Services (DHHS). Mental health: a report of the surgeon general. Rockville MD: substance abuse and mental health services administration, Center for Mental Health Services, National Institutes of health, National Institute of Mental Health; 1999.
46. Blasinsky M, Goldman H, Unutzer J. Project IMPACT: a report on barriers and facilitators to sustainability. Adm Policy Ment Health 2006;33:718–29.
47. Spitzer RL, Kroenke K, Williams JB, et al. A brief measure for assessing generalized anxiety disorder: the GAD-7. Arch Intern Med 2006;166:1092–7.
48. Lecrubier Y. Widespread under recognition and undertreatment of anxiety and mood disorders: results from 3 European studies. J Clin Psychiatry 2007;68: 36–41.
49. Ayers CR, Sorrell JT, Thorp SR, et al. Evidence-based psychological treatments for late-life anxiety. Psychol Aging 2007;22:8–17.
50. Thorp SR, Ayers CR, Nuevo R, et al. Meta-analysis comparing different behavioral treatments for late-life anxiety. Am J Geriatr Psychiatry 2009;17:105–15.
51. Wetherell JL, Lenze EJ, Stanley MA. Evidence-based treatment of geriatric anxiety disorders. Psychiatr Clin North Am 2005;28:871–96.
52. Andrade C. Psychopharmacology. In: Bhugra D, Ranjith G, Patel V, editors. Handbook of psychiatry: a South Asian perspective. New Delhi: Byword Publishers; 2005. p. 517–52.
53. Rollman BL, Belnap BH, Reynolds CF, et al. A randomized trial to improve the quality of treatment for panic and generalized anxiety disorders in primary care. Arch Gen Psychiatry 2005;2:1332–41.
54. Lauderdale SA, Sheikh JI. Anxiety disorders in older adults. Clin Geriatr Med 2003;19:721–41.
55. Department of Health. Impact assessment of the National Dementia Strategy. 2009. Available at: www.dh.gov.uk/en/Publicationsandstatistics/Publications/PublicationsPolicyAndGuidance/DH_094058?IdcService=GET_FILE&;dID=183502&Rendition=Web. Accessed October 3, 2012.
56. McKeith IG, Dickson DW, Lowe J, et al. Diagnosis and management of dementia with Lewy bodies. Third report of the DLB consortium. Neurology 2005;65: 1863–72.
57. Torke AM, Holtz LR, Hui S, et al. Palliative care for patients with dementia: a national survey. J Am Geriatr Soc 2010;58:2114–21.
58. Steffens DC, Maytan M, Helms MJ, et al. Prevalence and clinical correlates of neuropsychiatric symptoms in dementia. Am J Alzheimers Dis Other Demen 2005;20:367–73.
59. Craig D, Mirakhur A, Hart DJ, et al. A cross-sectional study of neuropsychiatric symptoms in 435 patients with Alzheimer's disease. Am J Geriatr Psychiatry 2005;13:460–8.

60. Fischer DC, Ladowsky-Brooks R, Millikin C, et al. Neuropsychological functioning and delusions in dementia: a pilot study. Aging Ment Health 2006;10:27–32.
61. Chiu MJ, Chen TF, Yip PK, et al. Behavioral and psychologic symptoms in different types of dementia. J Formos Med Assoc 2006;105:556–62.
62. Kaufer DI, Cummings JL, Christine D. Effect of tacrine on behavioral symptoms in Alzheimer's disease: an open label study. J Geriatr Psychiatry Neurol 1996;9:1–6.
63. Kales HC, Valenstein M, Kim HM, et al. Mortality risk in patients with dementia treated with antipsychotics versus other psychiatric medications. Am J Psychiatry 2007;164:1568–76.
64. Vahia I, Bankole A, Reyes P, et al. Schizophrenia in later life. Aging Health 2007; 3:383–96.
65. Howard R, Rabins PC, Seeman MV, et al. Late-onset schizophrenia and very-late-onset schizophrenia-like psychosis: an international consensus. Am J Psychiatry 2000;157:172–8.
66. Desai AK, Seraji M, Redden M, et al. Schizophrenia in older adults. How to adjust treatment to address managing patients' changing symptoms, comorbidities. Curr Psychiatr 2010;9:23–8.
67. Cohen CI, Vahia I, Reyes P, et al. Schizophrenia in later life: clinical symptoms and social well-being. Psychiatr Serv 2008;59:232–4.
68. Sadock BJ, Sadock VA. Kaplan and Sadock's synopsis of psychiatry: behavioral sciences/clinical psychiatry. 10th edition. Philadelphia: Lippincott Williams &Wilkins; 2007.
69. Substance Abuse and Mental Health Services Administration (SAMHSA). Results from the National Survey on Drug Use and Health: national findings. Rockville (MD): U.S. Department of Health and Human Services, SAMHSA, Office of Applied Studies; 2007. NSDUH Series H-32, DHHS Publication N. SMA 07–4293.
70. Savage SR. Addiction in the treatment of pain: significance, recognition and management. J Pain Symptom Manage 1993;8:265.
71. Carlat DJ. The psychiatric interview-a practical guide. 3rd edition. Philadelphia: Lippincott, Williams & Wilkins; 2012.
72. Eliason MJ. Identification of alcohol-related problems in older women. J Gerontol Nurs 1998;24:8–15.
73. Fingerhood M. Substance abuse in older people. J Am Geriatr Soc 2000;48: 985–95.
74. Adams SL, Waskel SA. Late onset of alcoholism among older Midwestern men in treatment. Psychol Rep 1991;68:432–4.
75. Morgan B, White D, Wallace A. In: Melillo K, Houde S, editors. Geropsychiatric and Mental Health Nursing. Boston: Jones & Bartlett; 2005. p. 199–200.
76. Brust JC. Neurologic disorders related to alcohol and other drug use. In: Ries RK, Freeman DA, Miller SC, et al, editors. Principles of addiction medicine. 4th edition. Philadelphia: Lippincott Williams and Wilkins; 2009. p. 1049–56.
77. Masters S. The alcohols. In: Katzung BG, editor. Basic and clinical pharmacology. 8th edition. New York: Lange Medical Books/McGraw-Hill; 2001. p. 382–94.
78. Saitz R. Medical and surgical complications of addiction. In: Ries RK, Freeman DA, Miller SC, et al, editors. Principles of addiction medicine. 4th edition. Philadelphia: Lippincott Williams and Wilkins; 2009. p. 945–67.
79. Atkinson RM. Treatment programs for aging alcoholics. In: Beresford TP, Gomberg ES, editors. Alcohol and aging. New York: Oxford University Press; 1995. p. 186.

80. Blow F. Treatment of older women with alcohol problems: meeting the challenge for a special population. Alcohol Clin Exp Res 2000;24:1257–66.

81. Rolland JS. In sickness and in health: the impact of illness on couples relationships. J Marital Fam Ther 1994;20:327–47.

82. Pachana N, Byrne G, Siddle H, et al. Development and validation of the geriatric anxiety inventory. Int Psychogeriatr 2007;19(1):103–14.

83. Andreescu C, Belnap BH, Rollman BL, et al. Generalized anxiety disorder severity scale validation in older adults. Am J Geriatr Psychiatry 2008;16(10):813–8.

84. Shankar KK, Walker M, Frost D, et al. The development of a valid and reliable scale for rating anxiety in dementia (RAID). Aging Ment Health 1999;3(1):39–49.

85. Schroder C, Johnson M, Morrison V, et al. Health condition, impairment, activity limitations: relationships with emotions and control cognitions in people with disabling conditions. Rehabil Psychol 2007;52(3):280–9.

86. Rinaldi P, Mecocci P, Benedetti C, et al. Validation of the five-item geriatric depression scale in elderly subject in three different settings. J Am Geriatr Soc 2003;51:694–8.

87. Borson S, Scanlan J, Brush M, et al. The Mini-Cog: a cognitive vital signs' measure for dementia screening in multi-lingual elderly. Int J Geriatr Psychiatry 2000;15:1021–7.

88. Schulman K, Shedletsky R, Silver I. The challenge of time. Clock drawing and cognitive function in the elderly. Int J Geriatr Psychiatry 1986;1:135–40.

89. Ewing J. Detecting alcoholism: the CAGE questionnaire. J Am Med Assoc 1984;252(14):1905–7.

90. Blow F, Brower K, et al. The Michigan Alcoholism Screening Test-Geriatric Version: a new elderly specific screening instrument. Alcoholism: Clinical and Experimental Research 1992;16:372.

Delirium in the Elderly Adult in Critical Care

Katheryne Tifuh Amba, MSN, CCRN, ACNP-BC, PhD (c)

KEYWORDS

- Delirium • Dementia • Elderly • Critical care

KEY POINTS

- Elderly patients with cognitive issues such as dementia have been shown to be at risk for delirium on admission into the intensive care unit.
- Dementia and delirium have similarities in that they both have a negative effect on mental status leading to memory impairment.
- Nonpharmacologic interventions such as discontinuation of restraints, Foley catheters, and loud alarm sounds from monitoring devices can help in decreasing delirium in the elderly.

INTRODUCTION

With the advances in sciences, the implementation of new technology in critical care, and the graying of the baby boomers; the critically ill demographic now encompasses a wide variety of patients. Elderly patients (aged >65 years) currently account for 42% to 52% of intensive care unit (ICU) admissions and for almost 60% of all ICU days.[1] Caring for the elderly in the ICU poses a special challenge because, as they age, neurologic changes affect their illnesses in addition to other comorbid conditions, making their management more complex. A plethora of neurologic issues abounds in the elderly adult population in critical care. An atypical presentation may involve a change in the elderly person's level of consciousness or some other acute cognitive changes that can be associated with alterations caused by infection, an imbalance of electrolytes, or drug toxicity. A thorough physical examination, with follow-up testing, must be conducted in order to accurately diagnose the origin of an elderly adult's neurologic changes. Age-related changes to the neurologic system, coupled with acute disorders and the ICU environment, may interact and increase a critically ill elderly adult's risk for postoperative cognitive dysfunction, falls, restraint use, oversedation, alterations in body temperature, and anorexia. These changes also increase the risk for one of the most commonly encountered disorders in the hospitalized elderly adult: delirium.[2]

The author has nothing to disclose.
Department of Neurosurgery, Barnes Jewish Hospital, One Barnes Plaza, St Louis, MO 63110, USA
E-mail address: Kta2761@bjc.org

Crit Care Nurs Clin N Am 26 (2014) 139–145
http://dx.doi.org/10.1016/j.ccell.2013.10.008
0899-5885/14/$ – see front matter © 2014 Elsevier Inc. All rights reserved.
ccnursing.theclinics.com

Research has shown that up to 45% to 70% of elderly adults admitted to an ICU experience an episode of delirium at some time during their hospital stay.[3]

Delirium

Delirium is acute confusion that develops over a short period of time and can fluctuate during the day and night. Delirium has more than 25 synonyms, including acute encephalopathy, septic encephalopathy, toxic psychosis, ICU psychosis, and acute confusional states.[4] Patients with delirium can have delusions and paranoia as well as motor changes. Delirium is a common and serious problem in hospitalized elderly patients.[5] For many years, critical care nursing and medical teams have considered delirium to be a benign problem, often considering that it will clear when the patient is out of the ICU.[6] Current research and publications now isolate delirium as a frequent complication in elderly adults in the ICU. Delirium has been associated with increased morbidity, mortality, and the length of stay in the hospital.[4,7–11] The American Psychiatric Association's Diagnostic and Statistical Manual, fourth edition[12] (DSM-IV) lists 4 key features that characterize delirium:

- Disturbance of consciousness with reduced ability to focus, sustain, or shift attention
- A change in cognition or the development of a perceptual disturbance that is not better accounted for by a preexisting, established, or evolving dementia
- The disturbance develops over a short period of time (usually hours to days) and tends to fluctuate during the course of the day
- Evidence from the history, physical examination, or laboratory findings that the disturbance is caused by a medical condition, substance intoxication, or medication side effect

The 4 subtypes of delirium are shown in **Table 1**.

CAUSES OF DELIRIUM

The causes of delirium are multifactorial.[13,14] Although pathophysiologic mechanisms of delirium remain unclear, current evidence suggests that disruption of neurotransmission, inflammation, or acute stress responses might all contribute to the development of this ailment.[3,15] A detailed discussion of the causes of delirium is beyond the scope of this article. A variety of neurologic conditions such as traumatic brain injury, electrolyte derangements, epilepsy, parasomnia, cerebrovascular accident, mental illness, urinary tract infection, alcohol intoxication, medication side effects, hypoglycemia, dementia,

Table 1 Four subtypes of delirium	
Type	**Symptoms**
Hyperactive delirium with high psychomotor activity	Patients are agitated, restless, disruptive, loud, and have a potential to inflict self-harm
Hypoactive delirium with low psychomotor activity	Patients are apathetic, withdrawn, have minimal interaction with care givers. They could be mistaken for having depression
Mixed delirium with features of both high and low psychomotor activities	Patient has traits of both hyperactive and hypoactive delirium
Delirium without psychomotor activity	Delirium with neither hyperactive nor hypoactive psychomotor activities

encephalopathy, and central nervous system infections have a high potential for the development of delirium. A change of environment from a familiar habitat into the ICU with numerous pieces of equipment, frequent assessments, and other iatrogenic effects can contribute to delirium.

It is important to perform a neurologic examination as soon as possible to determine neurologic dysfunction, establish a baseline, diagnose, and treat. Early assessments play an important role in identifying functional deficits and the patient's ability to function with activities of daily living.[16] **Table 2** presents the most common causes of delirium by using the acronym of MOVE, STUPID.[17]

Elderly patients with cognitive issues such as dementia have been shown to be at risk for delirium on admission into the ICU. There seems to be a fine line in differentiating elderly with dementia and those in delirium. Knowing some of the key differences between dementia and delirium can assist health care providers in screening and treating patients with acute confusional states. **Table 3** shows the differences between delirium and dementia.

Dementia and delirium have similarities in that they both have a negative effect on mental status leading to memory impairment, and carry a financial burden. Impaired memory with delirium is more prominent with patients in the hyperactive phase but, with dementia, it can be subtle and prominent in the late stages. Both conditions are costly to manage and treat and have an increased morbidity and mortality. These disease processes can provoke admission into critical care settings requiring specialized care.

CHALLENGES WITH DELIRIUM

Challenges to the caregivers center on establishing a mental status baseline. For instance, there may be concerns about whether the patient had dementia before

Table 2	
Most common causes of delirium	
M	Metabolic-B_{12} or thiamine deficiency, serotonin syndrome (elderly patients may not metabolize chemicals as well and as quickly as younger people, leading to deficiencies)
O	Oxygenation issues. Hypoxemia (the elderly have comorbidities that can put them at risk for hypoxemia. A decompensation of the respiratory or cardiac system can lead to fatalities related to hypoxemia)
V	Vascular causes. Cerebrovascular accidents, hypertensive emergencies, vasculitis, hyperviscosity, and myocardial infarction can lead to delirium
E	Electrolytes/endocrine dysfunction (hyponatremia is a common cause of confusion. Hypomagnesemia can fuel seizures, whereas hypokalemia causes arrhythmias)
S	Seizures/status epilepticus (in the elderly the impact of antiepileptic or injuries as a result of injury can be debilitating. Nonetheless, they account for confusional states)
T	Tumor, trauma, temperature, toxins (determining the problem with use of laboratory and radiological diagnostic exams is useful to isolate the cause of delirium)
U	Uremia, renal/hepatic dysfunction, urinary tract infections
P	Psychiatric, porphyria
I	Infection/inflammation (central nervous system and nonneurologic infections can manifest with delirium; eg, meningitis and encephalitis)
D	Drugs and alcohol (illicit drugs and prescription medications such as benzodiazepines have been shown to cause delirium as well as alcohol intoxication or severe alcohol withdrawal)

Table 3
Differentiating delirium and dementia

Dementia	Delirium
Chronic condition common in the elderly. Insidious onset. Months to years. Consciousness can be altered but patient is alert	Acute confused state. Onset precipitated by illness. Hours to months with fluctuations. Periods of alertness, hyperactive or hypoactive psychomotor activities or no psychomotor activity
Ongoing debilitating. Irreversible and patient unable to return to baseline	Can be treated and patient may return to baseline
Common in the elderly	Not age specific
Cause of disease involves decrease in brain cells, and Alzheimer is most common cause	The cause of delirium is multifactorial and it varies with each individual depending on the provoking and risk factors
Patients with dementia have the ability to stay focused, with periods of forgetfulness. Coherent speech except in late stages	Unable to stay focused. Confused, disoriented, and may cause self-harm unknowingly. Incoherent in hyperactive or hypoactive state

the escalation of the confusion or whether the patient suddenly became confused, as with individuals intoxicated with drugs or alcohol. By the time patients are admitted into the ICU, they have been consulted by other services. For instance, the patient may be examined in the emergency department (ED) initially and sent to radiology for imaging. This move may require transportation from one section of the hospital to another, necessitating some medications en route. By the time patients settle in the ICU, they have been through some sort of stress in addition to their presenting problem, which may make it challenging for clinicians to establish a baseline on the neurologic status.

Admission data from proxy sources such as family members or caregivers plays a crucial role in providing background information for the patient's history. Elderly adults in the postoperative phase may present special challenges because of sedation and poor metabolism of medications before admission into the ICU. Serial physical assessments and neurologic examinations are important to detect early deterioration. A spot or continuous electroencephalogram can provide key information to rule out subclinical seizure. Frequent monitoring for subtle signs of deterioration is highly recommended because prompt recognition allows caregivers to differentiate patients' symptoms.[18] Nonetheless, it is prudent to treat each patient as a unique entity to ensure best practices and better outcomes.

MANAGEMENT OF DELIRIUM

The screening and diagnosis processes in the elderly are challenging because of barriers to communicating effectively with the patient. Many elderly who are critically ill are voiceless,[19] partly because of the critical nature of their illness, especially those who are mechanically ventilated, a population that accounts for 70% to 80% of the population in critical care with delirium. Nurses play an important role because they frequently assess the patients and do screenings that may lead to the diagnosis of delirium. The original confusion assessment method of Ely and colleagues, in addition to the Confusion Assessment Method for the ICU (CAM-ICU) has shown validity and reliability among other scales to identify delirium in the ICU.[20,21] The CAM-ICU provides an algorithm to assess 4 key clinical criteria: acute onset and fluctuating course, inattention, disorganization thinking, and altered level of consciousness.[22]

Overall management of delirium is based on identifying and treating the underlying cause of the problem and ensuring a patient's safety in relation to the behavioral symptoms and challenges shown. The patient's chief complaint, history, and physical examination should be the driving factors for the diagnostic tests and examination. For instance, if the patient was unconscious as a result of a drug overdose, the administration of naloxone for narcotic overdose is a starting point to reverse the drug agent. If the underlying cause was seizure, electrolytes such as magnesium need to be supplemented. It is also prudent to initiate medications for seizure prophylaxis. Initial work-up for most elderly patients with delirium in critical care includes, but is not limited to, laboratory diagnostics of a complete blood count, complete metabolic panel, a toxicology screen, urinalysis, chest radiograph, head computed tomography (CT), an electroencephalogram if there are suspicions of seizure, and a lumbar puncture if infection is suspected.

Consideration of nonpharmacologic approaches and treatment of specific medical disorders always takes precedence. Life-threatening problems, such as hypoxia and hypoglycemia, and pain from acute diseases, such as myocardial infarction, require prompt attention.[23] Nonpharmacologic interventions such as discontinuation of restraints, Foley catheters, and loud alarms sounds from monitoring devices can help in decreasing delirium in the elderly. Allowing periods of rest with lights out and providing cluster care can play a positive role in treating delirium. Medications should be closely monitored for side effects that may provoke delirium. Early mobilization and implementing the Awakening and Breathing Coordination, Delirium Monitoring and Management, and early mobility (ABCDE) bundle are important factors to consider in managing delirium. The ABCDE bundle incorporates the best available evidence related to delirium, immobility, sedation/analgesia, and ventilator management in the ICU.[19] The bundle includes spontaneous awakening and breathing trial coordination, careful sedation choice, delirium monitoring, and early progressive mobility exercise.[6] Family presence, music, and animal therapy may enhance positive outcomes in patients with delirium. A typical delirium scenario is discussed later.

DELIRIUM CASE STUDY

Mr Jones, a 78-year-old widower, was found in the alley, half undressed and agitated, and was transported to the ED by paramedics. On arrival at the ED, his Glasgow Coma Scale was 9. He was unable to provide a reliable medical history and had no family members for support. Vital signs include a blood pressure of 190/100 mm Hg, pulse 112 beats per minute, respiration 28 breaths per minute, and temperature 38.0°C. On assessment by the nurse, his lungs sounded coarse, his abdomen was soft, and forehead laceration and bruises to knees and forearms were evaluated.

A CT scan of the head was performed and results revealed an intraparenchymal hemorrhage with a chronic subdural hemorrhage. The patient was admitted to the neurosurgical ICU. Two days after admission, Mr Jones became restless, was screaming, pulling out intravenous lines, and threatening to strike staff. He was placed on limb restraints and given more sedatives (lorazepam) for his restlessness and agitation. Family later confirmed the patient had a history of hypertension and dementia that made his medication compliance difficult, especially after his wife's death.

Mr Jones was admitted in the ICU for intraparenchymal hemorrhage. His hypertension was treated with intermittent intravenous hydralazine and an antibiotic was initiated for the urinary tract infection. Because of Mr Jones' age and history of dementia, he was at high risk for delirium. A neurosurgical consult was initiated to manage the intracranial hemorrhage. His delirium was associated with his urinary tract infection and he had an underlying condition of a cerebrovascular accident.

SUMMARY

Neurologic issues abound with the elderly in critical care settings. When the neurologic issues such as delirium are combined with the elderly patient's comorbidities, management may become a challenge to the health care providers and family members, leading to detrimental patient outcomes. A better understanding of the underlying causes and multiple neurologic and nonneurologic issues that can lead to delirium will assist clinicians to successfully manage elderly patients with delirium.

REFERENCES

1. Marik PE. Management of the critically ill geriatric patient. Crit Care Med 2006; 34(9):S176–82.
2. Balas MC, Casey CM, Happ MB. Assessment and management of older adults with complex illness in the critical care unit. AACN, GNEC Critical Care. Available at: http://hartfordign.org/uploads/File/gnec_state_of_science_papers/gnec_critical_care.pdf. Accessed September 16, 2013.
3. Balas MC, Deutschman CS, Sullivan-Marx EM, et al. Delirium in older patients in surgical intensive care units. J Nurs Scholarsh 2007;39(2):147–54.
4. Ely EW, Shintani A, Truman B, et al. Delirium as a predictor of mortality in mechanically ventilated patients in the intensive care unit. JAMA 2004;291(14):1753–62.
5. Saxena S, Lawley D. Delirium in the elderly: a clinical review. Postgrad Med J 2009;85:405–13.
6. Bell L. Delirium assessment and management. AACN practice alert. Available at: http://www.aacn.org/wd/practice/content/practicealerts/delirium-practice-alert.pcms. Accessed December 6, 2012.
7. Milbrandt EB, Deppen S, Harrison PL, et al. Costs associated with delirium in mechanically ventilated patients. Crit Care Med 2004;32(4):955–62.
8. Quimet S, Kavanagh BP, Gottfried SB, et al. Incidence, risk factors and consequences of ICU delirium. Intensive Care Med 2007;33(1):66–73.
9. Inouye SK. Delirium and other mental status problems in the older patient. In: Goldman L, Ausiello D, editors. Cecil medicine. 23rd edition. Philadelphia: Saunders Elsevier; 2007. Chapter 26.
10. Salluh JI, Soares M, Teles JM, et al. Delirium Epidemiology in Critical Care (DECCA): an international study. Crit Care 2010;14(6):210.
11. McNicoll L, Pisani MA, Zhang Y, et al. Delirium in the intensive care unit. Occurrence and clinical course in older patients. J Am Geriatr Soc 2003;51(5):591.
12. American Psychiatric Association. The American Psychiatric Association's diagnostic and statistical manual, 4th edition (DSM-IV). Arlington (VA): American Psychiatric Association; 2000.
13. Inouye SK, Charpentier PA. Precipitating factors for delirium in hospitalized elderly persons. JAMA 1996;275(11):852–7.
14. Inouye SK. Delirium in older persons. N Engl J Med 2006;354:1157–65.
15. Martins S, Fernandes L. Delirium in elderly people: a review. Frontiers in neurology. Available at: http://www.ncbi.nlm.nih.gov/pmc/articles/PMC3. Accessed November 19, 2012.

16. Hickey JV. The clinical practice of neurological and neurosurgical nursing. 6th edition. New York: Lippincott and Wilkins; 2009.
17. Le T, Mendoza M, Coffa D. First aid for the family medicine boards. 2nd edition. New York: McGraw Hill; 2012.
18. Devlin JA, Fong JJ, Howard EP, et al. Assessment of delirium in the intensive care unit; nursing practice and perceptions. Am J Crit Care 2008;17(6):555–65.
19. Balas MC, Eduard E, Burke WJ, et al. Critical care nurse's role in implementing the "ABCDE bundle" into practice. Crit Care Nurse 2012;32:35–47.
20. Ely EW, Inouye SK, Bernard GR, et al. Delirium in mechanically ventilated patients: validity and reliability of the confusion assessment method for the intensive care unit (CAM-ICU). JAMA 2001;286(21):2703.
21. Luetz A, Heymman A, Radtke FM, et al. Different assessment tools for intensive care unit delirium: which score to use? Crit Care Med 2010;38(2):409.
22. Lange JW. The nurse's role in promoting optimal health of older adults. Thriving on the wisdom years. Philadelphia: FA Davis; 2011.
23. Siegel MD. Management of agitation in the intensive care unit. Clin Chest Med 2003;24:713–25.

Oncologic Issues in the Older Adult in Critical Care

Roberta Kaplow, APRN-CCNS, PhD, AOCNS, CCRN

KEYWORDS

• Cancer • Oncology • Older persons • Geriatrics • Oncologic emergencies

KEY POINTS

• As the estimated number of older persons continues to increase, so does the estimated number diagnosed with cancer.
• The process of aging brings several physiologic changes that increase the risk of cancer as well as the comorbidities associated with a cancer diagnosis or its treatment.
• Older individuals are more likely to be admitted to the intensive care unit at some point during their disease trajectory.
• It is imperative for critical care nurses to be aware of the physiologic changes associated with aging, and the reasons for an older person with cancer to be admitted for prevention or treatment of oncologic emergencies.

INTRODUCTION

Even though people of all ages can receive a diagnosis of cancer, cancer is considered a disease of aging.[1,2] Between the years 2005 and 2009, the median age for a patient with a diagnosis of cancer (all sites) was 66 years. Almost 25% of patients were diagnosed between the ages of 65 and 74; 20.6% were diagnosed between the ages of 75 and 84; and 7.7% of patients were diagnosed at age 85 and older.[3] Comparing older adults with their younger counterparts, the incidence of cancer in patients of both genders and all races was 225.8 per 100,000 persons younger than 65 received a diagnosis of cancer while 2119.9 per 100,000 persons were 65 years and older.[3] More than 65% of all patients diagnosed with cancer were 65 years and older.[1,4,5]

With the projected increase in the older population comes an increase in the anticipated number of cancer cases up to 2050 (**Table 1**). Furthermore, the cancer survival rate has increased over the past 3 decades. Specifically, from 1975 to 1977 the cancer

Disclosures: None.
Conflict of Interest: None.
Department of Oncology, Emory University Hospital, 2184 Briarwood Bluff Northeast, Atlanta, GA 30319, USA
E-mail address: roberta.kaplow@emoryhealthcare.org

Table 1 Projected number of cancer cases for 2000 through 2050, based on projected census, United States			
Decade	Ages 65–74	Ages 75–84	Ages 85+
2010	416,896.8	309,509.2	129,969.7
2020	623,250.2	376,789	153,097.6
2030	754,156.6	577,297.7	203,943
2040	679,610.5	710,852.9	328,485.3
2050	719,310.7	654,560	447,394.1

Data from McEvoy LK, Cope DG. Caring for the older adult with cancer in the ambulatory setting. Pittsburgh (PA): Oncology Nursing Society; 2012. p. 1–7.

survival rate was 49%, indicating that this percentage of patients were alive 5 years after being diagnosed. From 1987 to 1989, the survival rate increased to 56%; and from 2001 to 2007 the survival rate climbed to 67%.[6,7] The increase in survivorship has been ascribed to advances in treatment and supportive care.[1,5]

Given the expected increase in the number of older people and the higher incidence of cancer in this group, it is increasingly likely that older patients with cancer will be admitted to the intensive care unit (ICU) for the prevention or management of complications of disease or treatments. It is therefore essential for critical care nurses to be mindful of the issues surrounding these individuals.[1] This article describes the pathophysiologic changes that occur with aging as they relate to cancer and cytotoxic therapies, implications related to drug therapy, and complications of treatment modalities as they relate to older person with cancer who may potentially be admitted to the ICU. Knowledge of these issues is essential for health care providers, so that they can face the complex challenges and optimize the outcomes of critically ill older persons with cancer.

PHARMACOLOGIC IMPLICATIONS OF AGING

Antineoplastic regimens have been increasing in complexity. Given the physiologic changes associated with aging (eg, hepatic and renal function), examination of the pharmacokinetics and pharmacodynamics of cancer therapies must take place. These changes may result in potentiated or decreased drug effects. Pharmacokinetics refers to how the body reacts to and copes with a drug. The 4 phases involved in pharmacokinetics are absorption, distribution, metabolism, and excretion.[8]

Absorption

Absorption, the first step in pharmacokinetics, occurs when a medication goes from its site of administration into the bloodstream. Many factors influence absorption, chief of which is how the medication is administered. Oral administration is the most complex modality, and requires several steps before it is absorbed. An oral medication must first be dissolved in gastric fluids. If a medication does not dissolve, it cannot be absorbed. It must then move to the site of absorption. Most absorption occurs in the duodenum of the small intestine, although some can occur in the stomach or large intestine.[9,10] Many conditions decrease drug absorption and prolong the drug effect; for example, drug metabolism in the liver is delayed and renal function is decreased in patients with hypothyroidism.[6] An example of the impact of gastrointestinal changes includes the development of oral mucositis, which may result in an increase in the absorption of oral agents. Likewise, changes in the skin, fat, or both may affect the absorption of topical agents.[11]

Distribution

Distribution is the second phase of pharmacokinetics, during which medication is delivered from the bloodstream to the target tissues where it will exert therapeutic effects. The more blood flow an organ receives, the more medication will be distributed there. The heart, liver, and kidneys are highly vascular organs that can have a large amount of drug delivered to them.[8]

Increase in age is associated with a decrease in total body water and an increase in total fat. These physiologic changes will affect drug distribution in the body.[11] Increased age is also associated with a decrease in plasma proteins. If an antineoplastic drug that is highly protein bound is administered, it drug will be less bound to protein in an older person. This process results in a higher amount of circulating drug left unbound and available to be bound to receptors, leading to higher concentrations of available active drug in the body.[11] Older adults who have a decreased albumin level may have higher drug levels, which may result in increased toxicities. Low serum albumin levels may also lead to a higher peak concentration of certain antineoplastic agents (eg, ifosfamide).

Increases in total fat may result in decreased elimination of fat-soluble drugs. The decrease in body water may cause a decrease in distribution of water-soluble drugs. Administration of an average drug dose may result in increased toxicities.[11]

Increased age is also associated with a decrease in red blood cells. Older persons with cancer, anemia related to disease, or on chemotherapy may be at risk for changes in drug distribution if the drugs (eg, taxanes) are highly bound to red blood cells.[11]

Metabolism

Metabolism is the third pharmacokinetic phase, and refers to the metabolic breakdown of a drug.[11] Once medications have been absorbed into the bloodstream, they can be metabolized. Metabolism occurs mainly in the liver. Oral medications are absorbed directly into the hepatic portal circulation, which delivers the medications to the liver where they are metabolized. This process is referred to as first-pass metabolism. First-pass metabolism is capable of inactivating large amounts of medication. If not given orally, medication will not go through first-pass metabolism.[8]

Hepatic changes associated with aging can alter the rate or extent of drug metabolism, or both. If drugs are metabolized more slowly, drug exposure is longer and there is potential for an increased risk of adverse events. On the other hand, if drugs are metabolized more quickly, a decrease in therapeutic effect can be anticipated.[11] In older adults, drug metabolism is decreased.

Excretion

Excretion is the removal of medication from the body, for which the kidneys are primarily responsible. Drug can also be removed through the lungs, intestine, bile, sweat, or breast milk.[8] The decrease in renal blood flow associated with aging affects delivery of medications or their metabolites to the kidney, which can lead to a decrease in elimination by the kidney and an increase in the half-life of these agents. The latter effect can result in increased toxicities. One example noted in the literature is the use of methotrexate. This agent, used in the treatment of several cancers (eg, lymphoma, sarcoma) as well as nononcologic conditions, must be used cautiously in patients with decreased renal function, as significant toxicities can occur. When methotrexate is used in patients with arthritis, monitoring of liver enzymes is essential in identifying the development of nonalcoholic cirrhosis. Another drug that is commonly administered in the oncology and ICU settings is morphine sulfate. When administered to patients with impaired renal function, accumulation of the drug or its metabolite can occur.[11]

Pharmacodynamics

Pharmacodynamics is the study of the effects medications have on the body. It is important for nurses to understand this concept, thus to be able to effectively counsel patients about what to expect from their medications. It is also important to understand pharmacodynamics so that patients can be monitored for therapeutic response, lack of therapeutic response, or adverse effects.

One example of pharmacodynamics for older patients with cancer is the bone-marrow suppression effects of chemotherapy. The degree and duration of bone-marrow suppression may be increased in older persons.[11]

AGONISTS AND ANTAGONISTS

Drugs exert their actions on cells by binding with receptors. Receptors are proteins on cells where molecules can bind and elicit a response. Chemicals naturally present in the body act on cellular receptors. Neurotransmitters (eg, serotonin) and hormones (eg, testosterone) are examples of endogenous (produced within the body) molecules that act on cellular receptors. Medications also act on cellular receptors to cause a response within the body.

When a medication is taken, it can either mimic a response that occurs in the body or block a response from occurring. A drug is referred to as an agonist if it mimics a response in the body. An agonist stimulates a response by activating receptors. Antagonists stop certain physiologic responses from happening.

DRUG INTERACTIONS

There is an increased risk of drug-drug interactions in older adults. Because of the physiologic changes associated with aging, patients with cancer may have several comorbidities requiring several medications to be taken. One study on polypharmacy with oncology pharmacists identified 12 clinically significant potential drug-drug interactions with oral antineoplastic agents and commonly used medications. Drug-drug interactions can lead to adverse clinical outcomes, particularly in oncology, because of the narrow antineoplastic index of oral agents and the high risk of additional medications prescribed for age-related organ dysfunction. Not all drug-drug interactions can be predicted, and those that are predictable are not always avoidable. However, increased awareness of the potential for these interactions will allow health care providers to minimize the risk by choosing appropriate drugs and monitoring for signs of interactions.

Complex regimens increase the risk of nonadherence. Patients who are on multiple medications, either for cancer treatment or as therapy for comorbid conditions, have to navigate the complexity of integrating the new cancer treatment into their lifestyle and current medication regimen, which can pose additional risks of medication and/ or food interactions. For example, a woman with advanced or metastatic breast cancer with tumors that overexpress HER2 may receive treatment with lapatinib (Tykerb) and capecitabine (Xeloda). She needs to take lapatinib once a day, 1 hour before a meal or 1 hour after a meal, whereas the capecitabine should be taken twice daily with food or within 30 minutes of eating.

ADVERSE DRUG REACTIONS

An adverse drug reaction is a reaction from the drug that is undesirable, unintended, and may not be well documented in the literature. It occurs within the normal dosage range of the drug. Older patients are often susceptible to adverse drug reactions because they may not metabolize or excrete medications as quickly as their younger counterparts. With age, the liver decreases in size and some hepatic enzyme activity is lost. There is also decreased hepatic blood flow, and first-pass metabolism can be diminished. As a result, older patients do not metabolize medications as effectively. Kidney size, glomerular filtration rates, and tubular secretion rates decrease. There are fewer nephrons available for drug excretion. Geriatric patients may also not drink enough fluids to maintain adequate hydration, further reducing renal blood flow. These factors decrease the amount of drug excreted in the urine. Reduction of liver and kidney function may cause an increase in serum drug concentrations, which increases the likelihood of side effects and possible toxicity. Based on these physiologic changes, in addition to the associated changes in drug pharmacokinetics and pharmacodynamics, drug doses in the geriatric patient are often lower than normal, and dosing intervals are extended. Polypharmacy is another identified contributor to increased vulnerability to adverse drug reactions in older persons.[8,11]

THE OLDER PATIENT WITH CANCER IN THE INTENSIVE CARE UNIT

As the number of older patients with cancer and any number of comorbidities and who are receiving antineoplastic therapies increases, the need for admission to the ICU is likely to increase also. Contributing to the need for ICU admission in this group of patients is the physiologic changes associated with aging, namely the age-associated weakening of the immune system. Older patients with cancer may be admitted to the ICU for several reasons. Admitting diagnoses that have been reported include respiratory failure, septic shock, hemodynamic instability, need for vasopressor administration or mechanical ventilation, renal dysfunction, bloodstream or intraperitoneal infection, or renal failure.[12–16]

Stages IIIB and IV non–small cell lung cancer (NSCLC) is another reported reason for admission to the ICU. In one study, patients with NSCLC who were older than 65 years were admitted to the ICU with respiratory, cardiac, or neurologic complications of the disease or treatment, sepsis, or renal failure. The patients with sepsis had the highest mortality rate. For these patients, the 90-day hospital mortality was 71% and the 1-year mortality rate was 90%.[17]

Several studies have been conducted to evaluate the outcomes of older patients with cancer who have been admitted to the ICU. Results of these studies have not been consistent. Overall survival has been reported to improve slightly over the past few years,[18] and has been variable depending on the reasons for ICU admission, cancer diagnosis, and acuity. Overall survival has ranged from 21.8% to 40%.[15,19] In one study, in which older patients had a lower survival rate, factors associated with a higher mortality rate in older patients with cancer included a higher severity of illness, uncontrolled cancer, the number of organ failures, and presence of a serious comorbidity.[20] In another study, older patients (≥75 years and older) had twice the mortality rate of their younger counterparts. The older patients in this study had an impaired level of consciousness, higher severity of illness, and either an infection on admission to the ICU or an ICU-acquired infection.[16]

Recommendations based on the study data included admitting patients for whom cancer treatment is available following ICU discharge[15]; not using age, underlying cancer diagnosis, or both as potential predictors of poor outcomes of an ICU admission, as some older patients may realize some benefit from an ICU admission[12,13,20,21]; and not admitting patients who have undergone a stem cell transplant and who require mechanical ventilation.[18]

Patients with cancer, in general, may also be admitted to the ICU for the prevention, early recognition, or management of 1 or more oncologic emergencies. Some of these potentially life-threatening conditions related to cancer-treatment modalities or the disease itself include increased intracranial pressure, cardiac tamponade, spinal cord compression, tumor lysis syndrome, sepsis/febrile neutropenia, superior vena cava syndrome, disseminated intravascular coagulation, syndrome of inappropriate secretion of antidiuretic hormone, and hypercalcemia of malignancy. Each of these oncologic emergencies is defined in **Table 2**.

Table 2
Oncologic emergencies

Oncologic Emergency	Definition
Increased intracranial pressure	Increased pressure within the skull related to expanding tumor volume and the production of associated cerebral edema, which results in a change in neurologic functioning
Cardiac tamponade	Severe compromise of the heart's ability to fill and pump, owing to an excessive accumulation of fluid, blood, or both in the pericardial sac; this results in an increase in pericardial pressure, a decrease in ventricular expansion and diastolic filling, and hemodynamic instability
Spinal cord compression	A neurologic emergency resulting from direct tumor invasion into the epidural space or outside the spinal cord
Tumor lysis syndrome	A life-threatening oncologic emergency characterized by metabolic abnormalities (ie, hyperkalemia, hyperphosphatemia, hyperuricemia, and hypocalcemia) that may lead to acute renal failure and multiple organ dysfunction syndrome
Sepsis	Infection plus 2 or more criteria of systemic inflammatory response syndrome (ie, temperature $\leq 36°C$ or $\geq 38°C$; heart rate ≥ 90 beats/min; respiratory rate ≥ 20 breaths/min; white blood cell count $\geq 12,000/\mu L$ or $\leq 4000/\mu L$, or >10% immature neutrophils)
Superior vena cava syndrome	Compression of the superior vena cava by tumor or enlarged nodes. It may also be caused by an internal obstruction of the vessel by thrombus
Disseminated intravascular coagulation	A complex systemic thrombohemorrhagic disorder involving the generation of intravascular fibrin and the consumption of coagulation factors and platelets. The resultant clinical condition is characterized by intravascular coagulation and hemorrhage
Syndrome of inappropriate secretion of antidiuretic hormone	Unregulated production of antidiuretic hormone that results in increased water retention by kidneys. The increased total body water and moderate expansion of plasma volume equates to water intoxication, resulting in a decrease in serum sodium to <135 mEq/L
Hypercalcemia of malignancy	Elevation of serum calcium to >12 mg/dL. The hypercalcemic state interferes with sodium and water reabsorption, leading to polyuria

Data from Refs.[22–25]

SUMMARY

As the estimated number of older persons continues to increase, so too does the estimated number diagnosed with cancer. The process of aging brings several physiologic changes that increase the risk of cancer as well as the comorbidities associated with a cancer diagnosis or its treatment. Older individuals are therefore more likely to be admitted to the ICU at some point during their disease trajectory. It is therefore imperative for critical care nurses to be aware of the physiologic changes associated with aging, and the reasons for an older person with cancer to be admitted for prevention or treatment of oncologic emergencies.

REFERENCES

1. Cope DG. Cancer and the aging population. In: Cope DG, Reb AM, editors. An evidence-based approach to the treatment and care of the older adult with cancer. Pittsburgh (PA): Oncology Nursing Society; 2006. p. 1–11.
2. Payne J. Research issues and priorities. In: Cope DG, Reb AM, editors. An evidence-based approach to the treatment and care of the older adult with cancer. Pittsburgh (PA): Oncology Nursing Society; 2006. p. 13–40.
3. Surveillance Epidemiology and End Results. Projected number of cancer cases for 2000 through 2050 based on projected census population estimates and age-specific cancer incidence rates, SEER and NPCR areas as reported by NAACCR, 1995-1999. Available at: http://seer.cancer.gov/report_to_nation/1973_1999/datapoints/figure5.pdf. Accessed September 7, 2012.
4. Alkekruse SF, Kosary CL, Krapcho M, et al. SEER cancer statistics review. Available at: http://seer.cancer.gov/csr/1975_2007. Accessed September 7, 2012.
5. McEvoy LK, Cope DG. Caring for the older adult with cancer in the ambulatory setting. Pittsburgh (PA): Oncology Nursing Society; 2012. p. 1–7.
6. American Cancer Society. Cancer facts and figures. Atlanta (GA): Author; 2012.
7. Merenda C. How far has the war on cancer come in the past 40 years? ONS Connect 2012;27(6):20.
8. Tarnowski A. Principles of pharmacology. In: Kaplow R, Hardin SR, editors. Pharmacology nursing essentials. Boston (MA): Jones and Bartlett, in press.
9. Aldred EM. How do drugs get into cells?. In: Aldred EM, editor. Pharmacology. A handbook for complementary healthcare professionals. London: Churchill Livingstone; 2008. p. 123–8.
10. Rang HP, Dale MM, Ritter JM, et al. Rang & Dale's pharmacology. 6th edition. London: Churchill Livingstone; 2007.
11. Schwartz RN. Pharmacologic issues. In: Cope DG, Reb AM, editors. An evidence-based approach to the treatment and care of the older adult with cancer. Pittsburgh (PA): Oncology Nursing Society; 2006. p. 91–102.
12. Chen TT, Peng MJ, Wu CL. Do elderly patients with non-hematologic malignancies have a worse outcome in the ICU? Int J Gerontol 2009;3:209–16.
13. Ferra C, Marcos P, Misis M, et al. Outcome and prognostic factors in patients with hematologic malignancies admitted to the intensive care unit: a single-center experience. Int J Hematol 2007;85:195–202.
14. Kew A, Couban S, Patrick W, et al. Outcome of hematopoietic stem cell transplant recipients admitted to the intensive care unit. Biol Blood Marrow Transplant 2006; 12:301–5.
15. Lecuyer L, Chevret S, Thiery G, et al. The ICU trial: a new admission policy for cancer patients requiring mechanical ventilation. Crit Care Med 2007;35: 808–14.

16. Vosylius S, Sipylaite J, Ivaskevicius J. Determinants of outcome in elderly patients admitted to the intensive care unit. Age Ageing 2005;34:157–62.
17. Bonomi MR, Smith CB, Mhango G, et al. Outcomes of elderly patients with stage 3B-IV non-small cell lung cancer admitted to the intensive care unit. Lung Cancer 2012;77:600–4.
18. Bruennier T, Mandraka F, Zierhut S, et al. Outcome of hemato-oncologic patients with and without stem cell transplantation in a medical ICU. Eur J Med Res 2007; 12:323–30.
19. Rellos K, Falagas ME, Vardakas KZ, et al. Outcome of critical ill oldest-old patients (aged 90 and older) admitted to the intensive care unit. J Am Geriatr Soc 2006;54:110–4.
20. Soares M, Carvalho MS, Salluh JI, et al. Effect of age on survival of critically ill patients with cancer. Crit Care Med 2006;34:715–21.
21. Karamiou K, Nichols DJ, Nichols CR. Intensive care unit outcomes in elderly cancer patients. Crit Care Clin 2003;19:657–75.
22. Becker JU. Disseminated intravascular coagulation in emergency medicine. 2011. Available at: http://emedicine.medscape.com/article/779097-overview. Accessed September 7, 2012.
23. Bone RC, Balk RA, Cerra FB, et al. Definitions for sepsis and organ failure and guidelines for the use of innovative therapies in sepsis. The ACCP/SCCM Consensus Conference Committee. American College of Chest Physicians/Society of Critical Care Medicine. Chest 1992;101:1644–55.
24. Itano J, Taoka KN. Metabolic emergencies. In: Itano J, Taoka KN, editors. Core curriculum for oncology nursing. 4th edition. Philadelphia: Elsevier Saunders; 2005. p. 383–421.
25. Itano J, Taoka KN. Structural emergencies. In: Itano J, Taoka KN, editors. Core curriculum for oncology nursing. 4th edition. Philadelphia: Elsevier Saunders; 2005. p. 422–39.

Nursing Practice of Palliative Care with Critically Ill Older Adults

Joan E. Dacher, PhD, MS, BS, GNP

KEYWORDS

- Palliative care • Critically ill older adults
- Clinical practice guidelines for quality palliative care
- Palliative care nursing practice with critically ill older adults

KEY POINTS

- The goal of palliative care is to prevent and relieve suffering, regardless of the stage of the disease or the need for other therapies.
- The National Consensus Project Clinical Practice Guidelines for Quality Palliative Care set the standard for palliative care in all settings, across all ages.
- Nurses can take a leadership role in pain and symptom management, identifying patient preference for goals of care, enhancing communication, and facilitating the family meeting.

INTRODUCTION

An unintended consequence of longevity and the aging of the population is an increase in the numbers of older adults experiencing critical illness, high disease burden, and the increased likelihood of hospitalization, specifically a patient on a critical care unit. By 2030, 9 million Americans will be older than 85 years and will experience disability and chronic illness, an increase from 4.2 million in 2000. Medicare beneficiaries with 5 or more chronic conditions are the fastest growing segment of the Medicare population.[1] Questions emerge within the literature as to the appropriateness of intensive medical intervention for many elders, particularly in light of the poor survival rates and diminished functional outcome experienced by many.[2] Evidence indicates that physicians are inaccurate and overly optimistic in the prognosis of terminally ill patients.[3] Once admitted to the critical care unit, elderly patients may enter into a trajectory of technologically intensive care, and in the absence of clearly articulated choices (made available at the point of care within the critical care unit), patients and families may default to the medically intensive care at hand.

Research supports the view that most Americans are not aware of the availability of any options for advanced care.[1] However, options do exist. Palliative care is emerging

Department of Nursing, The Sage Colleges, 65 First Street, Troy, NY 12180, USA
E-mail address: dachej@sage.edu

Crit Care Nurs Clin N Am 26 (2014) 155–170
http://dx.doi.org/10.1016/j.ccell.2013.10.003
0899-5885/14/$ – see front matter © 2014 Elsevier Inc. All rights reserved.

as an alternative care paradigm for critically ill older adult patients in the critical care setting, one that may radically alter prevailing assumptions about the care delivered and received in the critical care unit. Critical care nurses are well positioned to take on a leadership role in reconceptualizing care in the critical care unit, and creating the space and opportunity for palliative care. The purpose of this article is to provide critical care nurses with information on the practice of palliative care with critically ill older adults in addition to evidence-based content and resources, allowing them to advocate for palliative care in their own work environments accompanied by the necessary resources that will support efficient implementation.

National Consensus Project for Quality Palliative Care

A conceptual framework for implementing palliative care into health care settings can be found within the Clinical Practice Guidelines for Quality Palliative Care (CPG) released by the National Consensus Project for Quality Palliative Care. Clinical practice guidelines for quality palliative care, third edition, 2013. Available at: http://www.nationalconsensusproject.org/Guidelines_Download2.aspx. Accessed May 1, 2013. By making these quality guidelines available, the likelihood that evidenced based palliative care will be provided in all settings, including critical care, is enhanced. The Guidelines embody the highest standard for palliative care practice across the continuum of care. Endorsed by The National Quality Forum this affiliation assures measurable quality indicators for practice and an important element of legitimacy in light of the evidence that supports the application of these standards across health care. With its emphasis on the interdisciplinary team and the inclusion of the need to include age-specific disciplines and specialties with the plan of care, these CPG are appropriate for application for care of critically ill older adults within the critical care unit.

DEFINITION OF PALLIATIVE CARE

For the purposes of this article the definition of palliative care put forth by the National Consensus Project is used. This definition is contemporary and makes explicit the scope of support and services that are the necessary for the delivery of quality palliative care. Among other definitions of palliative care that are frequently encountered is that of the World Health Organization which is similar in spirit and intent. According the National Consensus Project:

> The goal of palliative care is to prevent and relieve suffering and to support the best possible quality of life for patients and their families, regardless of the stage of the disease or the need for other therapies. Palliative care is both a philosophy of care and an organized, highly structured system for delivering care. Palliative care expands traditional disease-model medical treatments to include the goals of enhancing quality of life for patient and family, optimizing function, and helping with decision making, and providing opportunities for personal growth. As such, it can be delivered concurrently with life-prolonging care or as the main focus of care.[4(p6)]

It is worth noting that palliative care is often thought to be a proxy term for hospice, and that the differences between the two are not well recognized or understood. Though different, there is a relationship between them. In understanding the two terms relative to each other, palliative care can be understood as the umbrella concept, the overarching philosophy that addresses care for individuals with severe and life-threatening illness, over the entire course of that illness, regardless of prognosis and expected length of life. Hospice refers to an organization that provides care for individuals at the end of life. The hospice insurance benefit sets the parameters for the extent and duration of care. Within the United States, to qualify for the hospice insurance benefit a medically determined prognosis of 6 months of life or less must be in place.[5] The differences between the two are significant and critical to issues of utilization of palliative care services. When patients misunderstand the term palliative care to mean only end-of-life care, they may be less willing to investigate and ultimately accept palliative care services and all it offers, particularly if they believe it means giving up treatment and they are not yet ready to do so. It is worth noting that palliative care is generally not covered by health insurance, thereby creating a significant barrier to care.

Palliation for Critically Ill Older Adults

Overall, older adults (persons ≥65 years) comprise more than 50% of all patient-days in the intensive care unit (ICU). Strong evidence indicates that adults who receive care in a critical care unit experience low rates of survival and, if they do survive, they experience significant functional morbidity: however, predicting outcomes-based comorbidities and prior health events is inexact.[2] Numerous studies indicate that survival and functional outcomes for older patients are worse than those for younger cohorts. A retrospective study of critically ill patients in the ICU who received cardiopulmonary resuscitation after a first cardiopulmonary arrest revealed that the overall rate of survival to discharge was 15.9%.[6] Age (≥65 years), along with nonwhite race and mechanical ventilation, were identified as being associated with lower survival. Patients who required pressors and experienced a cardiopulmonary arrest in an ICU were half as likely to survive to discharge.

Gershengorn and colleagues[7] identified similar outcomes for individuals who underwent cardiopulmonary resuscitation in the ICU. In an epidemiologic study of elderly patients in the United States who received cardiopulmonary resuscitation between 1992 and 2005, 18.3% of patients survived to hospital discharge. Another study found that for individuals in the ICU who experience cardiac arrest with pulseless electrical activity, there were no improvements in survival between 2000 and 2005. In another study, overall mortality rates among oldest-old (≥90 and older) ICU patients was higher than for younger adult patients, but not sufficiently high to make a case against admitting patients aged 90 and older to an ICU.[8] Overall, more than 1 in 5 deaths in the United States occurs in the ICU.[9]

In light of the strength of these data, there is evidence to support that many factors influence the likelihood of an older adult's survival after hospitalization in a critical care unit. In 2007 the American Association of Critical Care Nurses and the National Gerontological Nursing Association endorsed an evidence-based document that provides guidance for the care of the older adult with complex illness in the critical care unit.[10] The complex interactions that occur as a result of hospitalization within the critical care unit contribute to a poor outcome. Treatment decisions in this setting should not be driven by consideration of age alone. There is a confluence of risk and factors to which older adults are susceptible and which are associated with unfavorable outcomes, and these can be mitigated through targeted nursing interventions to promote the best possible outcome. This approach includes the recognition that it may be necessary to prepare patients and their families for the end of life, which may occur within the ICU, or a transfer that may be required to another hospital unit or outside of the acute care setting. Nurses who practice in the critical care setting are well positioned to influence the end-of-life care for older adults through the implementation of a patient-focused, team-based palliative care approach.

Integral to this discussion are the ethical and sociopolitical issues that arise from the increasing numbers of critically ill elders who are treated in the critical care setting.

Trends support that these numbers will increase in the future.[11] A prime question is that of resource allocation and the justification for the expenditure of scarce health care dollars on a small percentage of the population (those receiving care in critical care units), many of whom experience low survival rates. This concern is driven by the increase in the use of critical care by Medicare beneficiaries, along with the increase in cost to Medicare, primarily because of increased utilization.[12] Palliative care has proved to be effective at decreasing the costs associated with hospitalization (for individuals with live discharges as well as among those with hospital death) and, concomitantly, increasing quality of care and life with more effective pain and symptom management.[13] The potential reduction in health care costs will address many of the issues associated with effective utilization of health care resources.

Of the many ethical issues surrounding the care of critically ill older adults and end-of-life care in the critical care unit are those confronted by the nurses themselves, especially when caring for vulnerable elders. In a setting where curative care dominates, nurses are tasked with the job of coordinating and managing the work of sustaining life with complex equipment and medications, and providing support to patients and families who have hopeful expectations under the most tenuous of circumstances. In a study of moral distress among critical care nurses, Elpern and colleagues[14] identified that nurses are dissatisfied and experience distress in their practice in the critical care setting. The highest levels of distress occurred when nurses believed they were providing futile medically aggressive care. As the health professional who is most consistently with the patient, it is the nurse who witnesses disagreement and variation in approaches to care among physicians, and evasive behavior on the part of physicians when communicating with family members. These factors, along with dealing with angry family members and families not understanding the term life-sustaining measure, have been regarded as obstacles to providing end-of-life care and a source of distress.[15] The role of patient advocate for appropriate end-of-life care, in circumstances where nurses' actions are unlikely to influence outcome, is yet another source of moral distress, contributing to burnout.[16] As a profession, nursing embraces concepts of relief of pain and suffering, holistic care, engaging family in care, and promoting patient autonomy. The inability to provide all of these in the critical care setting is a source of frustration for nurses,[17] and contributes to the ethical dilemmas confronted by the nurses who are providing care to critically ill older adults. Each of these factors could be diminished or even eliminated with the implementation of palliative care in the critical care unit.

STANDARDS FOR PALLIATIVE CARE IN THE CRITICAL CARE UNIT

Although the essential purpose of the critical care unit (sustaining life), along with the use of highly complex medical intervention and technology, may suggest that it is an inappropriate environment in which to offer palliative care, increasingly this is not the case. As the place of death for increasing numbers of older adults in particular, the delivery of palliative care within medically intensive settings is increasingly accepted practice, and the recognition of the need is increasing. Differences do exist across hospitals; it is not yet a presence across all acute care settings, and the sophistication and expertise of the care is not yet consistent.[18,19] The dissemination and implementation of palliative care practice, research, and education is critical to assuring that quality palliative care is available in all acute care settings. Both the National Hospice and Palliative Care Organization (NHPCO) and the Center to Advance Palliative Care (CAPC) are the standard bearers in bringing this quality to all hospitals and into critical care settings in particular.

The NHPCO asserts that palliative care is the right of all patients, and issued a call-to-action position statement on access to palliative care in the critical care setting.[9] The document calls for a standard of care in critical care that would require palliative care be available for all patients; care providers in the setting would be responsible for developing the knowledge and skills necessary to provide the care. This approach is not viewed as specialty care but as care that is essential to and integrated in the routine practice of critical care. A consensus statement issued by the American College of Critical Care Medicine addresses the transition in care from cure to comfort that occurs when medically intensive care is no longer appropriate, as happens with so many critically ill older adults.[20] These recommendations (**Box 1**) complement the National Consensus Project for Quality Palliative Care Guidelines.

The CAPC initiative, Improving Palliative Care-ICU (IPAL-ICU), advocates for quality domains for palliative care in the ICU, similar to those put forth by The National Consensus Project and NHPCO.[21] In the monograph *Evaluation of ICU Palliative Care Quality*, the investigators cite the findings from various studies, including focus groups conducted with recovered ICU patients, families of patients, and families of patients who had died while in the ICU, highlighted as support for the IPAL-ICU initiative. These participants identified the need for timely, clear, and compassionate communications from clinicians; clinical decision making that is focused on patient preferences; care that promotes dignity, comfort, personhood, and privacy; and the ability for families to stay close to patients. Clinicians themselves highlighted the need for emotional support and organizational support for continuity of care. These recommendations become the basis for establishing measures for performance improvement to assure best clinical practices. In light of the high volume of critical care days dedicated to critically ill older adults and the outcomes associated with such care, the recommendations to improve critical care by implementing palliative care and supporting quality initiatives to assure a good outcome presents a singular opportunity to better meet the end-of-life care needs of this population.

SUCCESS OF IMPLEMENTING PALLIATIVE CARE IN CRITICAL CARE

Findings from the IPAL-ICU Project suggest 2 possible models for implementing palliative care in the critical care unit, the consultative model and the integrative model.[22]

Box 1
American College of Critical Care Medicine recommendations for palliative care

- Patient-centered and family-centered care and decision making
- Resolving conflict on end-of-life decision
- Communication with families
- Ethical principles relating to withdrawal of life-sustaining treatment
- Withdrawing life-sustaining treatment
- Symptom management in end-of-life care
- Considerations at the time of death
- Research, quality improvement, and education
- Needs of the interdisciplinary team

Data from Truog R, Campbell M, Curtis R, et al. Recommendations for end-of-life care in the intensive care unit: a consensus statement by the American College of Critical Care Medicine. Crit Care Med 2008;36(3):953–63.

The consultative model involves hospital-based palliative care consultants on the unit, particularly with the patients most at risk for poor outcomes; elderly patients especially are likely candidates for their care. Criteria are generally established to identify the triggers that indicate the need for a consultation. The integrative model takes the approach of entrenching palliative care into the practice of the unit; all team members become knowledgable in palliative care practice and all patients receive care through a lens of palliative care, although there may be subgroups of patients for whom care is targeted. Both models use the domains of the National Consensus Project to guide design and function. There is evidence to support both models, and advantages and disadvantages to each. The decision of which to implement, or to choose a hybrid model, is a function of multiple factors:

- Presence of a hospital-based palliative care team with availability to provide services to the ICU and capability for collaboration with critical care team
- Receptiveness of members of the critical care team to change in practice and develop knowledge in palliative care
- Agreement among all stakeholders in favor of particular model characteristics
- Evaluation of baseline data including prior resource utilization on the unit, patient outcomes, and targeted efficiencies such as implementation of a patient plan of care within an appropriate time frame or a decrease in the number of treatments with low efficacy

There is strong evidence that implementing palliative care in this setting will result in changes in care that will be of benefit to all patients, and older patients in particular.[23,24] Among the outcomes most significant to the care of elders are increases in the numbers of: (1) individuals disconnected from ventilators, (2) recommendations for pain medications and symptom management, (3) advanced directives completed, (4) Do Not Resuscitate orders completed, and (5) patients who are referred to and enrolled in a hospice.

NURSING PRACTICE OF PALLIATIVE CARE

Critical care nursing has long recognized the imperative of responding to the needs of patients at the end of life. In 1999 the Nursing Leadership Consortium on End-of-Life-Care (Consortium) was organized to develop a strategic blueprint and move forward the profession's commitment to improve care at the end of life. The American Association of Critical Care Nurses (AACN) participated in this effort and, along with 22 other nursing specialty organizations, endorsed an agenda to improve end-of-life nursing care.[25]

The National Consensus Project

In addition to offering a comprehensive definition of palliative care, the report of the National Consensus Project, the Clinical Practice Guidelines for Quality Palliative Care, offers a consistent approach to palliative care that can be applied across all settings for all populations of any age and with a wide range of diagnoses.[4] The CPG identify 8 domains of quality palliative care, with specific guidelines and criteria that describe the essential elements of care and the evaluation of the quality of the care delivered. With the addition of extensive bibliographies and domain-specific exemplars, the CPG translate easily to provide comprehensive care and support of critically ill older adults and their families. The work of the nurse in this setting is such that the role becomes the linchpin for effective palliative care of the elderly. Consistent nursing presence with patient and families, ongoing communication with other team members, and continuous proximity to the point of care ideally situate nurses to be at the forefront of efforts to implement palliative care. The historic role of the nurse as advocate also lends itself to this concept. **Table 1** provides an overview of the 8 domains of palliative care, focal areas of the guidelines and criteria, and nursing activity in the critical care unit to support implementation of the guidelines.

The Physical Environment of the ICU

These guidelines are comprehensive but not specific to the critical care unit. Within this setting, among the other variables that warrant attention is that of environment. The physical environment of the unit is a problematic and challenging setting in which to offer quality palliative care. Among the environmental characteristics regarded as essential to quality end-of-life care are privacy, proximity to home, the cleanliness and homeliness of the environment, specific environmental inadequacies including excessive noise, proximity to sounds of pain and discomfort from other patients, limited waiting-room space, and level of cleanliness.[26] Though perhaps not as important as quality of care itself, all of these factors contribute to appropriate care.

Several of these characteristics are particularly critical to older adults. Older critically ill patients are at risk for delirium in the critical care unit, and excessive noise contributes to this risk. Family members who are elderly themselves may be more sensitive to the noise, and for those with hearing deficits there is the risk of impaired communication. Because hearing aids augment all sound, it is difficult to discriminate and selectively attend to specific sounds. The clutter of the environment may contribute to an increase in falls for older patients and their visitors. The issue of proximity to home is particularly critical to older family members who may be reliant on public transportation or costly cab rides to visit, or who may have impaired vision and are unable to drive at night. This last concern is not a nursing matter per se, but is something nurses need to be aware of so that they can offer the support of other team members to provide assistance.

In any given critical care environment, there are limitations to the extent to which the physical environment can be altered. Given this constraint, there are actions the nurse can take to proactively assess the patient and family members to ameliorate the impact of these limitations. Screening for delirium from the day of admission allows for early identification and intervention, including altering the environment to the fullest possible extent. The Intensive Care Delirium Screening Checklist is an appropriate tool that is brief and easily implemented.[27] Exploring patient and family preferences on admission, to identify potentially stressful and calming environmental features, will allow the nurse to enhance the environment to the extent required. With elderly family and friends, it is useful to ask about transportation issues and offer to bring in other team members (eg, social workers) who are able to address such issues. The issue of privacy can be addressed through working with the entire staff to develop guidelines for providing privacy on the unit and incorporating them into regular practice. Conducting conversations with elderly family members with hearing impairment should take place in a quiet environment to optimize communication. This location also reduces the stress of being in a noisy environment and the fear of not hearing, which are liable to increase stress and make conversations and decision making more difficult.

The End of Life National Education Consortium (ELNEC), a national initiative to promote palliative care, provides nurses (among others) with an opportunity to receive ELNEC training using a train-the-trainer model. Among the specialty areas offered to Registered Nursing are separate in-depth population-specific courses on critical care and geriatrics.[28] For nurses who work in critical care settings and are

Table 1
Application of national consensus guidelines to care of critically ill older adults

Domain	Focal Areas of Guidelines and Criteria	Nursing Skills and Activities
Structure and processes of care	Assessment of patient and family is comprehensive and interdisciplinary	Knowledge of essential elements of palliative plan of care
	Plan of care is timely, based on input of patient, family, providers, etc	Assures functional baseline status of patient is known
	Assessment is ongoing	Facilitates communication to assures that patient and family preferences for goals of care are known and documented
	Treatment decisions are based on goals of care including patient and family choice	When patient is unable to communicate, works with family and significant others to identify patient's values and make that voice known
	Changes in care over time are documented	Is competent in the practice of palliative care and is a recognized member of the palliative care team
	Specialist-level palliative care is delivered by an interdisciplinary team	Assumes role as patient and family advocate
	Care is provided in the environment most preferred by the patient and family	Supports transition from curative care to palliative care, assures that patient and family are the center of all support/interventions
		Is able to practice within the structure of an interdisciplinary collaborative team
		Communicates with all members of palliative care team to assure consistency in approach to care and assure that the patient's preferences and goals of care are met
Physical aspects of care	Pain and symptom management are evidence-based and disease-specific	Provides comprehensive pain/symptom assessment that addresses patient status and needs
	Interdisciplinary team includes professionals skilled in symptom control	Understands patterns of disease progression in the elderly
	Pain and symptoms are assessed regularly	Uses evidence-based tools to assess pain and symptoms in the elderly
	Pain and symptom management is safe, timely, and ongoing, to a level that is acceptable to patient and family	Uses evidence-based tools to assess pain in elders with cognitive impairment
	Barriers to pain management are recognized and addressed	Addresses family questions and concerns regarding use of analgesics and narcotics, and provides education as needed
	Patient and family understanding of disease processes is assessed	Educates patient (when possible) and family about symptom management
	Relief of distress is comprehensive and includes a variety of approaches	Applies knowledge of physiologic changes of aging to pain and symptom management
		Applies knowledge of pain management including common disease-specific syndromes and their manifestation in the elderly
		Applies knowledge of symptom management of dyspnea, depression, dementia, anxiety, and terminal restlessness associated with dying process
		Uses knowledge of the risks for and causes of delirium in older adults to minimize likelihood of occurrence
		Understands age-related changes and how they affect physical status of aging
		Uses appropriate management of pain in the elderly associated with diagnostic and treatment procedures

Psychological and psychiatric aspects of care	Psychological status is assessed, interventions are evidence-based Psychiatric issues are addressed Family education is available A range of therapies is available: pharmacologic, nonpharmacologic, complementary Specialists deliver age-appropriate care A grief/bereavement risk assessment and intervention are available Support is developmentally, culturally and spiritually appropriate	Understands the developmental needs of older adults and builds this into the plan of care as appropriate Has knowledge of and uses evidence-based grief assessment tools Addresses previously existing mental health issues Uses a variety of techniques to communicate with nonverbal patients and individuals who are cognitively impaired Facilitates culturally appropriate support for grief and bereavement of all family members Recognizes the difference between uncomplicated and complicated grief Recognizes the difference between grief and depression in older adults Knows when to appropriately seek the services of other team members to provide psychological support Seeks information regarding particular age cohort–related life experiences of the older adult that could affect psychological status
Social aspects of care	Comprehensive interdisciplinary assessment is available Social needs of patients and families are identified Care plan is developed Assessment is developmentally appropriate Social care plan reflects and documents patient and family preferences	Assures that social assessment is comprehensive and age-appropriate, and addresses all aspects of patient and family life before illness and hospitalization Applies knowledge of the developmental needs of older adults to developing and implementing care plan Identifies all members of the patient's social unit including nonfamily members Identifies the way to include family members in care as appropriate, including older individuals Uses a flexible approach to care to engage family as a social unit and meet patient and family needs
Spiritual, religious, and existential aspects of care	Interdisciplinary team includes professionals skilled in assessing and response to spiritual/existential issues Regular and ongoing assessment is conducted Interventions are based on care needs, goals consistent with patient and family values Pastoral care and palliative team facilitate access to spiritual community, groups, and clergy Palliative care team facilitates and advocates for religious and spiritual rituals as directed	Understands the difference between spirituality and religiosity as applied to palliative care nursing Has knowledge of spiritual assessment tools Provides evidence-based spiritual assessment that is appropriate for use with an older patient Engages pastoral care as a source of consultation or support as necessary Seeks expert knowledge of unique spiritual and religious rituals and practices if unknown

(continued on next page)

Table 1
(continued)

Domain	Focal Areas of Guidelines and Criteria	Nursing Skills and Activities
Cultural aspects of care	Palliative care team assesses and attempts to meet cultural needs of patient and family Cultural needs and concerns are addressed in plan of care Communication is respectful of cultural preferences Communication occurs in a language the patient and family understands, with all reasonable efforts made to use interpreter services Recruitment and hiring practices reflect the cultural diversity of the community	Provides evidence-based cultural assessment tool Seeks information of culture-specific rituals and practices related to care of the sick and dying Uses or advocates for the use of interpreters as needed Seeks expert knowledge of unique cultural rituals and practices if unknown Knowledge of ethnogeriatrics or care for older adults from culturally diverse populations
Care of the imminently dying patient	Signs and symptoms of impending death are recognized, documented, and communicated appropriately to patient, family, and staff End-of-life concerns and expectations are discussed openly and in a culturally and developmentally appropriate manner Plan of care is revised to meet needs of patient and family Transition to hospice will be introduced Education on signs and symptoms of death is provided to family	Uses knowledge of indicators of terminal stage of life and imminent death, including those that are disease-specific, to provide education to family Has the skill to and engages patient and family in honest discussion about disease status and end-life-issues using therapeutic communication techniques Advocates for and introduces transition to hospice; has knowledge of hospice services and hospice referral system Engages family to plan for death so that patient and family preferences are addressed Provides active support for family during the process of death Provides culturally appropriate care of the body after death

| Ethical and legal aspects of care | Patient goals, preferences, and choices are respected in keeping with state and federal law and standards of medical care and from the basis for the plan of care

Interdisciplinary team includes professionals expert in ethical, legal, and regulatory medical decision making

Patient's or surrogate's wishes from the basis for care plan

Evidence of patient preference is sought

Advanced care planning is promoted

In the event the patient is unable to communicate preferences, the team advocates for evidence of previously expressed wishes, honoring known preferences | Works with all members of interdisciplinary comprehensive care team to provide uniform approach to end-of-life discussions

Advocates for patient's end-of-life preferences

Uses evidence-based tools for assessing goals of care

Has basic knowledge of state-specific paperwork and requirements for end-of-life decision making

Has knowledge of hospital process for end-of-life decision making

Recognizes ethical conflict and dilemmas, and uses appropriate resources to seek resolution

Recognizes that goals of care evolve over time and reassesses as appropriate

Recognizes one's own stress and the stress of fellow staff members as a result of working in a high-intensity environment, and seeks appropriate support |

contemplating implementing palliative care services, the availability of ELNEC creates an opportunity to identify a champion who will then support program development through the dissemination of expert knowledge. The training is designed to support this type of program development. The curriculum focuses on core areas of palliative care nursing: Nursing Care at the End of Life; Pain management, Recommended Competencies; Communication; Loss, Grief, Bereavement; and Preparation for and Care at the Time of Death. These core modules are intentionally aligned with the 8 domains identified as part of the National Consensus Project quality guidelines. As a nationally and internationally recognized initiative, ELNEC training and dissemination within a given nursing setting is in indication of significant commitment to implementation of the highest level of quality palliative care. This initiative is recommended to support program development.

Communication and Family Meetings

Effective communication is in integral component of palliative care, involving patients, family, and other members of the care team. The complexity of end-life-care is such that it is difficult to easily characterize the qualities of effective communication, especially with regard to patients and families. What nurses may take for granted as a straightforward and essential exchange can be perceived as harsh and uncaring. Given the setting and context, there is likelihood that much of what is shared will be perceived as bad news. The discussion of prognosis, cessation of treatment, and preferences for end-of-life care is inherently painful for patients, families, and nurses. The pace of critical care is also a significant impediment. Communication depends on being attentive to words and the nuances of language and gestures or body language; subtleties may be lost if there is a lack of time. Without sufficient time to spend with family and patients, it is difficult to establish the necessary relationship that effective communication requires.

The ability to use good communication skills under difficult circumstances is essential to the practice of critical care nursing in this setting. Patients often see health care professionals as having the responsibility to introduce the end-of-life discussions. In a study of health care professionals on their perceptions of the transition of patients in heart failure to palliative care, nurses were generally perceived as more approachable than physicians, in part because they have more physical presence. In addition, a physician's lack of confidence in discussing sensitive issues was identified as a driver of ineffective communication, thereby strengthening the need for the nurse to take on this responsibility.[29]

Some strategies to enhance nurse-patient-family-team communication include adequate staffing, so that nurses have sufficient time to spend with family members and talk. This approach may involve prioritizing patient assignments so that patients at the end of life are cared for by nurses they and the family are familiar with, and decreasing the workload for a nurse who is caring for someone at the end of life. Providing private spaces for the family to speak with staff also promotes discussion and disclosure that is less apt to take place in more public spaces.

Effective use of the family meeting to establish goals of care based on patient and family values and preferences, with the involvement of all team members, offers many benefits. This type of group communication increases the potential for greater understanding among all team members of the plan, with a greater likelihood that it will be followed. The family receives the benefit of the knowledge of all team members, and knows that everyone has discussed and has heard consistent information. Nelson and colleagues[30,31] developed a toolkit for conducting family meetings in the ICU. The 3 tools, termed the Family Meeting Planner, the Family Meeting Guide, and the Family

Meeting Documentation Template, optimize communication, provide an effective framework to deal with difficult conversations, and can be used for performance improvement, particularly for a communication outcome. The use of an integrated interdisciplinary team to care and support older adults is a standard of care in gerontology, particularly so when working with those who are critically ill, and is a recommendation of the National Consensus Guidelines.

Palliative Care Nursing Practice with the Elderly

Successful palliative intervention for critically ill older adults is predicated on nursing practice founded on a synthesis of the disciplines of gerontology and geriatric nursing, critical care nursing, and palliative care. Although the principles of palliative care are readily applied to all age groups, they align well with essential elements of care for the elderly, which are to promote care that is holistic, comprehensive, and individualized, engages family, promote autonomy, and include patients in decision making to the fullest extent possible. Care for older adults is different from that for patients of other ages. Health status is likely to be more complex in the presence of multiple

---

Box 2
Recommended resources

- AACN Self-Assessment: Palliative and End-of-Life Care.

http://www.aacn.org/wd/palliative/content/palandeolinfo.pcms?menu=

- AACN Promoting Excellence in Palliative and End-of-Life Care e-Learning Course.

http://www.aacn.org/wd/palliative/content/palandeolinfo.pcms?menu=

- Center for the Advancement of Palliative Care IPAL-ICU Initiative.

http://www.capc.org/ipal/ipal-icu

- Hartford Institute for Geriatric Nursing Try This Series.

http://hartfordign.org/resources/try_this_series/

- Hartford Institute for Geriatric Nursing Consult GeriRN series.

http://consultgerirn.org/

- Robert Wood Johnson Foundation: Promoting Excellence at End-of-Life.

http://www.aacn.org/WD/Palliative/Content/PalAndEOLHome.content?menu=Practice

- ELNCEC.

http://www.aacn.nche.edu/elnec

- ELNEC On-Line Resources.

http://www.aacn.nche.edu/elnec/elnec-web-resources

- Confusion Assessment Method for the ICU.

http://www.mc.vanderbilt.edu/icudelirium/docs/CAM_ICU_flowsheet.pdf,

http://www.mc.vanderbilt.edu/icudelirium/docs/ICDSC.pdf

- Assessment of Spirituality in Older Adults: FICA Tool.

http://consultgerirn.org/uploads/File/trythis/try_this_sp5.pdf

- EthnoGeriatrics and Cultural Competence for Nursing Practice.

http://consultgerirn.org/topics/ethnogeriatrics_and_cultural_competence_for_nursing_practice/want_to_know_more comorbidities and complex medical histories. Moreover, physiologic changes associated with aging require that treatment and interventions are adjusted accordingly. The elderly patient brings an intricate life story that influences the preferences for care in the face of critical illness and at the end of life. Ageism and lack of knowledge about the aging body may create a cultural context that may manifest itself in the care received at the end of life, creating a greater imperative for integrating knowledge from multiple disciplines to create an inclusive foundation of care. By utilizing resources from all disciplines, critical care nurses will be able to develop the necessary knowledge and skills. **Box 2** contains some recommended resources for the critical care nurse who desires to build knowledge to provide palliative care to older adults in the critical care setting and to support the implementation of more formalized palliative care in such a setting.

SUMMARY

Palliative care, like so much else in health care, is evolutionary. While there is strong evidence to support efficacy and desirable outcomes for its practice, changes in health care practice and policy, as well as questions related to finance and quality health outcomes, will further the ongoing discussion on maintaining currency with demands for and changes in care. The acceptance of palliative care services among all populations will likely increase over time, and it makes sense that this will also be the case with older adults. Critical care nurses are likely to further this end. When implementing palliative care in this setting, critical care nurses are the team members most likely to embrace it and express enthusiasm; unit physicians are slower to acknowledge the necessity or merit.[22] Evidence supports that these nurses recognize the need to move from a culture of medical discourse to one that makes relief of suffering the primary priority, welcoming a culture of care as it emerges from a culture of cure. The need to do this is well supported by the reality of the clinical outcomes of older patients who receive care on a critical care unit.

The maturity of palliative care as a discipline is such that there are ample resources available to guide nursing practice with critically ill older adults. These resources include clinical practice guidelines, end-of-life education for critical care nurses, technical assistance from the CAPC through the IPAL-ICU Project, the opportunity to designate a Critical Care ELNEC trainer, models for implementation, books, and journals.

Critical care nurses are well positioned to take on a leadership role in implementing palliative care. As evidenced in the literature, they already recognize the need, and are witnesses to the suffering that takes place. Nurses understand the burden imposed on patients and families by the absence of palliative care. In such situations nurses themselves experience negative consequences, including moral distress and burnout. As the team members most present with patients and families and the primary providers of care, critical care nurses excel at symptom management and providing continuity of care. The values of nursing are congruent with those of palliative care, so much so that the clinical practice of palliative care with all patients, and older adults in particular, is a natural progression of critical care nursing practice.

REFERENCES

1. Advance illness care: key statistics. In: Coalition to transform advanced care. 2012. Available at: https://docs.google.com/file/d/0B2Yr38cBOUqzUkhWLWJyZ25YQIU/edit?pli=1. Accessed February 10, 2013.

2. Nguyen YL, Angus DC, Boumendil A, et al. The challenge of admitting the very elderly to intensive care. Ann Intensive Care 2011;1(1):29.
3. Christakis NA. Extent and determinants of error in doctors' prognoses in terminally ill patients: prospective cohort study. BMJ 2000;320:469.
4. National Consensus Project for Quality Palliative Care. Clinical practice guidelines for quality palliative care, second edition. 2009. Available at: http://www.nationalconsensusproject.org/guideline.pdf. Accessed February 12, 2013.
5. About hospice and palliative care: what is hospice? National Hospice and Palliative Care Organization; 2013. Available at: http://www.nhpco.org/about/about-hospice-and-palliative-care. Accessed February 26, 2013.
6. Ehlenbach W, Barnato A, Curtis R, et al. Epidemiologic study of in-hospital cardiopulmonary resuscitation in the elderly. N Engl J Med 2009;361:22–31.
7. Gershengorn H, Li G, Kramer A, et al. Survival and functional outcomes after cardiopulmonary resuscitation in the intensive care unit. J Crit Care 2012;27: 421.e9–17.
8. Rellos K, Falagas ME, Vardakas KZ, et al. Outcome of critically ill oldest-old patients (aged 90 and older) admitted to the intensive care unit. J Am Geriatr Soc 2006;54:110–4.
9. Position statement on access to palliative care in critical care settings: a call to action. National Hospice & Palliative Care Organization; 2008. Available at: http://www.nhpco.org/sites/default/files/public/NHPCO_PC-in-ICU_statement_Sept08.pdf. Accessed February 8, 2013.
10. Balas M, Casey C, Happ M. Assessment and management of older adults with complex illness in the critical care unit. The National Gerontological Nursing Association; 2008. Available at: http://www.harfordign.org/uploads/File/gnec_state_of_science_papers/gnec_critical_care.pdf. Accessed February 8, 2013.
11. Jakob SM, Rothen HU. Intensive care 1980-1995: change in patient characteristics, nursing workload and outcome. Intensive Care Med 1997;23:1165–70.
12. Milbrandt EB, Kersten A, Rahim MT, et al. Growth of intensive care unit resource use and its estimated cost in Medicare. Crit Care Med 2008;36(9):2504–10.
13. Sherman DW, Cheon J. Palliative care: a paradigm of care responsive to the demand for health care reform in America. Nurs Econ 2012;30(3):153–66.
14. Elpern EH, Covert B, Kleinpell R. Moral distress of staff nurses in a medical intensive care unit. Am J Crit Care 2005;14(6):523–30.
15. Beckstrand R, Kirchhoff K. Providing end-of-life care to patients: critical care nurses' perceived obstacles and supportive behaviors. Am J Crit Care 2005; 14(5):395–403.
16. Robichauz CM, Clark AP. Practice of expert critical care nurses in situations of prognostic conflict at the end of life. Am J Crit Care 2006;15(5):480–9.
17. Davidson P, Introna K, Daly J, et al. Cardiorespiratory nurses' perceptions of palliative care in nonmalignant disease: data for the development of clinical practice. Am J Crit Care 2003;12(1):47–53.
18. Trossman S. Critical initiatives palliative care services complement not contradict ICU care. Am Nurse 2004;36(4):1, 7–8.
19. Bush H. The evolution of palliative care. Hosp Health Netw 2012;86(2):38–40, 50.
20. Truog R, Campbell M, Curtis R, et al. Recommendations for end-of-life care in the intensive care unit: a consensus statement by the American College of Critical Care Medicine. Crit Care Med 2008;36(3):953–63.
21. Nelson J, Brasel K, Campbell M, et al. Evaluation of ICU palliative care quality: a technical assistance monograph form the IPAL-ICU project. The Center to Advance

Palliative Care; 2010. Available at: http://ipal-live.capc.stackop.com/downloads/ipal-icu-evaluation-of-icu-palliative-care-quality.pdf. Accessed February 10, 2013.

22. Nelson J, Bassett R, Boss R, et al. Models for structuring a clinical initiative to enhance palliative care in the intensive care unit: a report from the IPAL-ICU Project. Crit Care Med 2010;38(9):1765–72.

23. O'Mahony S, McHenry J, Blank M, et al. Preliminary report of the integration of a palliative care team into an intensive care unit. Palliat Med 2010;24(2):154–65.

24. Curtis JR, Treece PD, Nielsen EL, et al. Integrating palliative and critical care evaluation of a quality-improvement intervention. Am J Respir Crit Care Med 2008; 178:269–75.

25. Report of the nursing leadership consortium on end-of-life care. Designing an agenda for the nursing profession on end-of-life care. 1999. Workshop report. Available at: http://www.aacn.org/WD/Practice/Docs/Designing_Agenda.pdf. Accessed February 17, 2013.

26. Brereton L, Gardiner C, Gott M, et al. The hospital environment for end of life care of older adults and their families: an integrative review. J Adv Nurs 2011;68(5): 981–93.

27. Bergeron N, Dubois MJ, Dumont M, et al. Intensive care delirium screening checklist: evaluation of a new screening tool. Intensive Care Med 2001;27(5): 859–64.

28. End-of-life nursing education consortium fact sheet. Available at: http://apps.aacn.nche.edu/ELNEC/factsheet.htm. Accessed February 17, 2013.

29. Green E, Gardiner C, Gott M, et al. Exploring the extent of communication surrounding transitions to palliative care in heart failure: the perspectives of health care professionals. J Palliat Care 2011;27(2):107–16.

30. Nelson J, Walker A, Luhrs C, et al. Family meetings made simpler: a toolkit for the intensive care unit. J Crit Care 2009;24:626.

31. Nelson J, Cortez T, Curtis JR, et al. Integrating palliative care in the ICU the nurse in a leading role. J Hosp Palliat Nurs 2011;13(2):89–94.

Index

Note: Page numbers of article titles are in **boldface** type.

Crit Care Nurs Clin N Am 26 (2014) 171–179
http://dx.doi.org/10.1016/S0899-5885(13)00111-1
0899-5885/14/$ – see front matter © 2014 Elsevier Inc. All rights reserved.

Moving?

Make sure your subscription moves with you!

To notify us of your new address, find your **Clinics Account Number** (located on your mailing label above your name), and contact customer service at:

Email: journalscustomerservice-usa@elsevier.com

800-654-2452 (subscribers in the U.S. & Canada)
314-447-8871 (subscribers outside of the U.S. & Canada)

Fax number: 314-447-8029

Elsevier Health Sciences Division
Subscription Customer Service
3251 Riverport Lane
Maryland Heights, MO 63043

*To ensure uninterrupted delivery of your subscription, please notify us at least 4 weeks in advance of move.

ELSEVIER

Printed and bound by CPI Group (UK) Ltd, Croydon, CR0 4YY

03/10/2024

01040390-0018